The GP Quiz Book 1

Detection and management of physical disease

Alick Munro

RADCLIFFE MEDICAL PRESS

© 1999 Alick Munro

Radcliffe Medical Press Ltd
18 Marcham Road, Abingdon, Oxon OX14 1AA

British Library Cataloguing in Publication Data
A catalogue record for this book is available from the British Library.

ISBN 1 85775 229 5

Typeset by Joshua Associates Ltd, Oxford
Printed and bound by Hobbs the Printers, Totton, Hants

Contents

Preface

Some of the best clinical teachers I had as a student and junior hospital doctor used to conduct their tutorials and ward rounds as quizzes. Sometimes the answers were unknown even to them, but the format stimulated thought, discussion and library searches. I used to think it unfortunate that only a small minority of the medical textbooks then available had quizzes on the subject matter as an appendix. Using them allows us to rapidly spot important gaps in our knowledge and direct our reading accordingly. Quizzes also help us to maintain interest in the subject.

When the postgraduate education allowance was introduced in 1990, I started producing quizzes from the content of the *British Medical Journal* and the *British Journal of General Practice*. Both of these journals carry peer-reviewed original research and authoritative reviews. Every 3 months, members of our Doctors' Reading Club earn their PGEA by filling out a quiz review based on recent material in these journals. I formulate the questions with a mind to drawing attention to those matters which came as important news to me, or which seem most likely to influence the thoughts of fellow GPs on how best to practise. Members return the quiz reviews for checking and scoring, and then receive them back with model answers to the factual questions and summaries of their answers to the debatable points contained in our newsletter.

The quiz reviews and the material from the newsletter have now been collated by topic for publication, and also to satisfy our members who required this format for ease of reference. This book is limited to the detection and management of physical disease, and because of this it has a preponderance of factual questions. It is anticipated that books on psychological, social preventative and management issues will follow.

How might readers use this book? It does not contain a comprehensive account of any topic. Many of the thought-provoking questions have been addressed by summarizing the points made by the authors of original articles and by members of our Doctors' Reading Club, and by adding comments of my own based on additional reading. The answers are perhaps not the last word on these open-ended subjects. However, the book is designed to be a stimulating read, concentrated on those matters most likely to affect how GPs work. It is suited to intermittent browsing, and sometimes that is all a GP has time for. However, I myself find it useful to have the text available as an *aide-memoire* in the consulting room.

Students, trainees and practitioners may find that this format helps them to identify and plug important gaps in their knowledge, and locate recent authoritative evidence for more detailed study.

I hope you will enjoy the book, and I would like to thank the contributors and editing staff at the journals and the members of Doctors' Reading Club whose writings have provided me with so much interest.

Dr Alick Munro MRCP MSc
April 1999

Doctors' Reading Club welcomes new members. As well as the quarterly quiz review, members air their own uncertainties and reflections on practice in our newsletter and receive feedback from their fellow members. The current subscription is £96 per year and an additional £90 per year if you require reprints of source articles.

Doctors' Reading Club
FREEPOST (TK1586)
Twickenham
TW1 1BR

ASTHMA

Aetiology and demographics

1 What factors in prenatal or early life experience may predispose to atopy?

BMJ. **314**: 987–8 (leading article)

2 Evidence from this study suggests that the following commonly exacerbate asthma:

a feather pillows

b furry pets

c a damp bedroom

d moving house.

BMJ. **311**: 1053–5 (original paper), 1069–70 (original paper)

3 What allergens might cause occupational asthma in the following groups?

a Flour millers (*2 points*)

b Laundry workers (*1 point*)

c Wood workers (*1 point*)

BMJ. **316**: 2997–9 (review)

4 A survey of 12–14 year old children in the UK reveals that 19.8% have had treatment with anti-asthma drugs in the past year and between 5% and 8% were experiencing moderate or worse symptoms which were currently poorly controlled. Which of the following were also findings from this project? (*True/False*)

- Prevalence is higher in urban areas.
- Prevalence is higher in native-born children.

BMJ. **316**: 1118–23 (survey report)

5 Children who wheeze after a viral infection of the respiratory tract are likely to be atopic. (*True/False*)

BMJ. **315**: 858–62 (trial report)

6 What proportion of women with asthma find that it gets worse just before their period?

BMJ. **314**: 1842 (citation)

7 Which insect in addition to the house-dust mite produces excreta which are allergenic to the airways? (*1 point*)

BMJ. **312**: 1630 (news item)

8 What factors may explain this research finding that use of a wood or coal stove as the main source of heating in a house is associated with a signific- antly lowered risk of bronchial hyper-responsiveness in children compared to use of gas, oil or other forms of central heating? (*3 or more points*)

BMJ. **312**: 1448–50 (research report)

9 A manual worker develops asthma.

a What substances might you enquire about when seeking to determine if he has had occupational exposure to an allergen or irritant? (*8 points*)

b What screening investigation might you undertake to check the possibility that the asthma is of occupational origin? (*2 points*)

BMJ. **313**: 291–4 (review article)

10 Patients who report asthma symptoms on a questionnaire but have not brought them to the attention of a doctor are:

a likely to constitute about what percentage of the practice list?

b likely to be concentrated in what subgroups of the population? (*3 points*)

Br J Gen Pract. **46**: 295–7

11 In this survey of patients taking repeat prescriptions for asthma treatments:

a what percentage suffered wheeze at least once per week?

b what percentage avoided mild exercise between attacks?

c what percentage were current smokers?

d what percentage had a poor inhaler technique?

BMJ. **304**: 361–4

Diagnosis and assessment

1 How often should a patient blow into a peak-flow meter at each time of recording, and what observation should he record?

BMJ. **302**: 738

2 **a** What improvement in peak flow 15 min after inhaling 400 mcg of salbutamol constitutes a positive response?

b Diurnal variability in peak flow is defined as

$$\frac{\text{highest PEF } - \text{ lowest PEF}}{\text{mean PEF}} \times 100$$

What is the minimum percentage diurnal variability that indicates asthma?

Br J Gen Pract. **46**: 193–7 (discussion paper)

3 In a child with a history of cough the following features are suggestive of long-term bronchial hyper-reactivity. (*True/False*)

a Cough is worse at night.

b Wheeze has been noted.

c Cough is accompanied by vomiting.

d History of dyspnoea.

Br J Gen Pract. **41**: 406–9

4 Which children with asthma may usefully have skin tests? (*2 points*)

BMJ. **306**: 1676–81

5 What social factors are associated with under-diagnosis of asthma in adolescents? (*5 points*)

BMJ. **316**: 651–4 (survey report)

6 The writer of this article suggests a stamp (reproduced below) to mark the record card when reviewing a patient with asthma. Would you like to suggest any refinements to the stamp?

BMJ. **311**: 1473–8 (research report)

```
┌─────────────────────────────────────────────────────────────┐
│                                                               │
│  Date:                      Asthma review                     │
│  ─────────────────────────────────────────────────────       │
│                                                               │
│                        Day        Night       Exercise        │
│  Symptoms:                                                     │
│                                                               │
│  Days unable to work/off school:                              │
│                                                               │
│  Beta-agonist use per day:                                    │
│                                                               │
│  ─────────────────────────────────────────────────────       │
│                                                               │
│  Smoking? Yes/No            Occupation:                       │
│                                                               │
│  Peak-flow rate:            Inhaler technique:                │
│                                                               │
│    – Actual                   – Good/Moderate/Poor            │
│                                                               │
│    – Expected best                                            │
│                                                               │
│    – Home range             Peak-flow meter? Yes/No           │
│                                                               │
│  Prophylaxis?                                                 │
│                                                               │
│  – Increase/Decrease Start/Stop                               │
│                                                               │
│  Self-management plan? Yes/No                                 │
│                                                               │
│  ─────────────────────────────────────────────────────       │
│                                                               │
│  Plan:                                                        │
│                                                               │
└─────────────────────────────────────────────────────────────┘
```

Self-management

1 'Education must be of potential benefit to asthma sufferers, but it is obviously difficult to determine the right level of information or how to impart it.' Which of the following formats seems appropriate for educating asthmatics in your practice? State two reasons for your policy.

- Routine consultation.

- Extended consultation.

- Consultation with practice nurse trained in asthma management.

- Group evening class for asthmatics or parents of asthmatics.

- Other (*describe*).

Br J Gen Pract. **41**: 224–6

2 Patients who are prescribed a policy for monitoring and flexible treatment for their asthma:

a require a peak-flow meter

b consult their GPs for emergency treatment of asthma less frequently thereafter.

BMJ. **301**: 1355–9

3 What information do you need on an asthmatic patient in order to devise a self-management plan for his or her condition? (*4 or more points*)

BMJ. **308**: 564–71, 1099–100

4 Most asthmatics find it difficult to perceive the severity of their current airflow obstruction as shown on their peak-flow recordings. What implications does this have for practice? (*3 or more points*)

BMJ. **307**: 422–4

5 The parents of a child with asthma request information on how to use their peak-flow meter. In what circumstances should they use it, and for what purposes? (*6 points*)

BMJ. **305**: 1128–9

6 What reduction in morning peak flow do you think should trigger:

a a doubling of dose of inhaled steroid for 2 weeks

b use of oral steroid for 2 weeks?

BMJ. **312**: 748–52 (research report), 762–5

7 What might an asthmatic do to reduce the content of irritant air pollutants in the public rooms of his or her house? (*3 or more points*)

BMJ. **312**: 1316 (review)

8 Why may synthetic pillows be more likely to provoke asthma than feather ones?

BMJ. **313**: 916 (research report)

9 Which dietary modifications appear likely to minimize chronic obstructive airways disease? (*6 points*)

BMJ. **310**: 75–6 (editorial)

10 Why does washing a spacer device for inhaled medication improve its performance?

BMJ. **314**: 1661–2 (leading article)

11 Small spacer chambers are as efficient as large ones for delivering the content of metered-dose inhalers. (*True/False*)

BMJ. **313**: 320 (news item)

12 Two puffs of bronchodilator delivered together into a spacer inhaler provide twice the dose that one puff does. (*True/False*)

BMJ. **306**: 1066

13 List three or more items of advice to parents of an asthmatic child using a home nebulizer to prevent over-dosage and unwise delay in seeking medical help.

BMJ. **302**: 1180–1, **302**: 1599–600

14 How can one tell when an anti-asthmatic aerosol canister no longer contains medication? (*1 point*)

BMJ. **307**: 726–7

15 What should be done to prevent asthmatics from running out of inhaled medication? (*3 or more points*)

Br J Gen Pract. **47**: 125

16 An asthmatic has been needing 15 mg prednisolone per day for over a year to control his asthma. What should he do if he develops diarrhoea and vomiting? (*3 points*)

BMJ. **306**: 1078

17 What advice do you give your asthmatics who require inhaled steroids on adaptation to a period of summer smog? (*3 points*)

BMJ. **309**: 619–20

18 This study found that parents tended to use bronchodilator aerosols for their toddlers at times that were unrelated to their reports of asthma symptoms, despite being aware that there was a timer device on the spacer tube which would be analysed by staff at the clinic. What strategies might help parents of asthmatic children aged under 5 years to use inhalers more effectively? (*2 or more points*)

BMJ. **310**: 1161–4

19 Children with asthma should increase their use of prophylactic drugs until their frequency of wheeze, persistent cough or requirement for bronchodilators declines to no more than three times per week. Is this a reasonable policy? Can you devise a better guideline for use of anti-asthma drugs for children? (*2 or more points*)

BMJ. **311**: 663–6 (review), 1065–9 (original paper)

20 The author suggests that parents of asthmatic children be given crisis packs of prednisolone to use in an emergency. What selection criteria would you use to identify suitable patients in whom to apply this policy? (*3 or more points*)

BMJ. **311**: 810 (letter)

21 What reasons may underlie this report that asthmatics who require major tranquillizers have a higher mortality from asthma than other asthmatics? (*2 or more points*)

BMJ. **312**: 79–81 (research paper)

22 What advice on treatment would you give the following patients with cough or wheeze?

a A 9-month-old baby has had nocturnal cough for the past week. She appears listless but has no abnormal physical signs. The same symptoms about 2 months ago did not respond to reassurance, a warm moist atmosphere and simple linctus, but subsided after about 2 weeks. (*2 points*)

b A 7-year-old boy gets nocturnal cough and wheeze for up to 2 weeks if he catches a cold. It has happened twice in the past year. He has used no anti-asthma medicines up to now. (*2 points*)

c A 65-year-old man of medium height who usually takes high-dose inhaled steroids twice daily and two puffs of bronchodilator if he gets wheezy has been wheezing for the past 12 h and is breathless and exhausted when you see him in the evening. He is much better after inhaling a nebule of salbutamol and one of beclomethasone, and his peak flow has improved from 150 to 220 L/min. His pulse rate is now 95 beats/min and his respiration rate is 18 breaths/min. (*3 points*)

BMJ. **306**: 776–82, 1131–2

Medical treatment

1 The latest UK guidelines on asthma management suggest the following:
(*True/False*)

a inhaled steroid treatment should be introduced gradually and stepped up

b long-acting beta-agonists should be introduced before long-term high-dose inhaled steroids

c sodium cromoglycate is the prophylactic of first choice in small infants.

BMJ. **314**: 315–16 (leading article)

2 The following guidelines on asthma management are supported by good evidence. (*True/False*)

a Two puffs of salmeterol 50 mcg are better than one.

b Salmeterol should be considered when overnight control of asthma is required.

c Increasing the frequency of use of inhaled steroids to four times per day may permit a lower total daily dose than doubling the dose that is taken twice daily.

BMJ. **312**: 762–5 (guidelines)

3 What dose of steroid given by what route is recommended by the British Thoracic Association for the treatment of acute asthma in adults if the peak-flow rate is in the range 40–74% of the predicted or best value?

BMJ. **301**: 1272

4 A 5-year-old asthmatic child, who is usually well controlled on maintenance treatment with beta-stimulant, steroid and cromoglycate by inhalation, occasionally develops severe asthma when he has a cold. What additional treatment can be provided at the start of a cold in order to prevent this?

BMJ. **302**: 948

5 A short course of prednisolone is contraindicated in an asthmatic with a proven peptic ulcer in the recent past. (*True/False*)

BMJ. **304**: 655

6 Intramuscular progesterone has been used successfully as a treatment for premenstrual asthma. (*True/False*)

BMJ. **302**: 1453

7 Short-term treatment with inhaled budesonide is associated with reduced bone growth. (*True/False*)

BMJ. **303**: 163–5

8 Children who wheeze after a viral infection of the respiratory tract: (*True/False*)

a obtain a statistically significant long-term benefit in FEV_1 from using beclomethasone dipropionate as Diskhaler 200 mcg bd

b obtain a statistically significant benefit in FEV_1 on stopping treatment with beclomethasone dipropionate as Diskhaler 200 mcg bd

c experience a statistically significant reduction in the frequency of respiratory symptoms with regular use of beclomethasone dipropionate as Diskhaler 200 mcg bd.

BMJ. **315**: 858–62 (trial report)

9 The following observations can be expected in adults with chronic obstructive airways disease on maintenance treatment with inhaled bronchodilators alone. (*True/False*)

a Over 1 year FEV_1 declines significantly more in patients treated four times daily with inhaled bronchodilators than in those treated intermittently on demand.

b The decline in FEV_1 is similar in patients with bronchitis and those with asthma.

c The decline is similar in patients treated with salbutamol and those treated with ipratropium bromide.

d Patients on intermittent on-demand treatment prefer salbutamol to ipratropium bromide.

BMJ. **303**: 1426–31, **304**: 121

10 What advantage does the Nebuhaler spacer tube have over the Volumatic?

Br J Gen Pract. **305**: 429–32

11 Large-volume spacer devices with aerosol canisters are more efficient than dry-powder devices for delivering inhaled drugs to the lung. (*True/False*)

BMJ. **305**: 598

12 A patient taking a 12-day course of prednisolone to treat an acute exacerbation of asthma should be tailed off the treatment gradually. (*True/False*)

*Br J Gen Pract.***43**: 222–3

13 Theophylline treatment: (*True/False*)

a may be useful in patients who do not respond adequately to beta-agonists

b plasma levels are directly related to dose in an individual patient

c erythromycin increases plasma levels

d cimetidine increases blood levels

e the dose of a delayed-release formulation can be based on assay in a plasma sample 12 h after dosing.

*BMJ.***305**: 1355–8

14 A 35-year-old asthmatic suffers nocturnal wheeze on one night in three and occasional daytime wheeze despite taking inhaled salbutamol on going to bed every night and at onset of symptoms. In this situation the following treatment regimes are justified:

a inhaled salmeterol on going to bed

b inhaled steroid twice daily – salbutamol on going to bed and at onset of wheeze

c inhaled steroid twice daily – stop salbutamol

d inhaled cromoglycate four times daily, with salbutamol on going to bed and at onset of wheeze.

*BMJ.***302**: 1166–7

15 Why may an H_2 antagonist help an asthmatic?

*BMJ.***306**: 1403–5

16 How can PACT data be used to determine whether a practice is making effective use of asthma treatments?

*BMJ.***307**:12671–3

17 Steroids from aerosol inhalers should always be delivered through a spacer device. Why?

*BMJ.***307**: 12671–3

18 An asthmatic has a salbutamol inhaler and a spacer device. How should he use them during and after an acute attack of asthma?

*BMJ.***307**: 12671–3

19 Why may a spacer device and face mask be unsuitable as a delivery system for bronchodilator aerosols for very small children?

BMJ. **306**: 1676–81

20 A postmenopausal female asthmatic requires 15 mg prednisolone per day to control her condition. What additional or alternative treatments might improve her prognosis?

BMJ. **305**: 413–15

21 When treating asthma in children: (*True/False*)

a acaricides can be generally recommended

b salmeterol is best used only in conjunction with an anti-inflammatory agent

c combining an inhaled steroid with cromoglycate gives added benefit

d in high doses budesonide has less effect on the adrenal than does beclomethasone dipropionate

e the Turbohaler needs less suction to trigger it than does the Diskhaler/ Rotahaler.

BMJ. **310**: 1522–7

22 You are going to introduce treatment with an ACE inhibitor to a patient with asthma. What precautions will you take?

BMJ. **307**: 8–21

23 Prolonged use of inhaled steroids will permanently alter the long-term course of childhood asthma. (*True/False*)

BMJ. **308**: 1584–5

24 What percentage of the dose of anti-asthma remedies can be expected to be deposited in the lung using the following inhalation techniques?

a Metered-dose inhaler – patient with poor technique.

b Metered-dose inhaler – patient with good technique.

c Metered-dose inhaler with spacer chamber.

d Dry-powder inhaler – fast inhalation.

e Dry-powder inhaler – slow inhalation.

Br J Gen Pract. **45**: 683–7 (review)

25 How might you go about conducting a trial of response to steroids in a patient with suspected asthma?

BMJ. **316**: 150 (letter)

26 If children with acute asthma are treated with intravenous salbutamol, what reduction in the duration of requirement for nebulized salbutamol would you expect?

BMJ. **314**: 397 (news report)

27 By how much do high-dose inhaled steroids increase the risk of developing glaucoma?

BMJ. **314**: 697 (news report)

28 What ocular danger may be associated with combined use of ipratropium and salbutamol in a nebulizer?

BMJ. **304**: 40

29 Montelukast: (*True/False*)

a blocks the asthmatic response to non-steroidal anti-inflammatories

b blocks the asthmatic response to exercise in cold, dry air.

BMJ. **316**: 1257–8 (leading article)

ANSWERS

Aetiology and demographics

1 Being the first born, suffering relatively few infectious illnesses in early life, and avoiding contact with other infants and children are factors that cause Th lymphocytes to be expressed as Th2 rather than Th1 lymphocytes, and this predisposes to atopy.

   Suspicion that fetal undernutrition in the latter stages of pregnancy may predispose to atopy is also under investigation.

2 a False – in fact changing to a synthetic pillow may increase the risk.

   b True – owning furry pets at the time of the asthmatic's birth and during their teenage years appears to increase the risk by 70–100%.

   c False – unless mould is also present, when the risk is approximately doubled.

   d True.

3 a Flour, grain mites.

   b *Bacillus subtilis* in detergent.

   c Plicatic acid in resin of pine and western red cedar.

4 a False – if anything the prevalence in metropolitan areas is lower than that in rural areas.

   b True – the prevalence appears to be higher in native-born children, but this may be the result of a reporting bias.

5 True – about half of the children recruited to this study were atopic.

6 Two-fifths.

7 The cockroach.

8 Different populations – wood or coal stoves were mainly found in rural areas. Houses with wood or coal stoves are kept cooler, thus inhibiting the house-dust mite. Wood and coal stoves improve ventilation.

9 Paint, animal proteins, grain, glue, resins, wood dust, soldering flux, enzymes. A 3-hourly record of peak flow for a whole week.

10 a Possibly about 7%.

   b Women and moderate to heavy smokers.

11 a 49%.

   b 4%.

   c 14%.

   d 22%.

Diagnosis and assessment

1 The best of three recordings.

2 **a** 60 L/min.

   b 15%.

3 **a** True.

   b False.

   c False.

   d False.

4 Those aged over 5 years, off steroids, and in contact with an avoidable allergen. However, skin allergy does not correspond closely to airway allergy, although it may have more predictive value for allergens causing rhinitis.

5 The results from this survey from Denmark suggest the following: low physical activity, high body mass, serious family problems, passive smoking, female sex.

6 The stamp produced by the original authors had space for matters which are subject to change, such as symptoms, peak-flow rate, disturbance of daily activities, use of treatments, and management advice, as well as matters that are likely to be permanent or semi-permanent characteristics, such as smoking, best peak-flow rate, availability of spacer device and peak-flow meter, smoking status, occupation, and efficiency of use of aerosol inhalers.

   The two types of information might best be stored on either side of a record card. To the list of variable factors members suggested adding hospital admissions for asthma, last use of oral steroid, and whether the review was initiated by the doctor or the patient.

   To the list of permanent or annually reviewed characteristics members suggested adding use of flu vaccine, pneumococcal vaccine, FEV_1, and known precipitants of attacks and, for children, their height and weight and centile values.

Self-management

1 Information is most likely to be accepted at a time when the patient is asking for it. A check-list of important points discussed with the patient could be used as a basis for the discussion. Items can be ticked when they are discussed and the check-list kept in patients' notes. Information booklets for patients can be used to reinforce the message. A nurse can provide the service but will require training. Group evening classes might be useful, but the level of attendance at these is often disappointing.

2 **a** False – the results are just as good if monitoring is based on symptoms.

   b True – the reduction is by about 75%.

3   Every asthmatic requires information on how to monitor his or her asthma and adjust the medication that has been prescribed. However, common sense would dictate that only those who experience frequent and sustained episodes of limited airflow will benefit from basing their treatment on peak-flow readings. Obviously they must also be willing and able to use a meter effectively, both to determine their own best readings and to determine the readings they obtain during an attack. Patients who can predict their peak flows from how they feel, and those who can predict when asthma will affect them from exposure to allergens or infections, may have less need for a meter. The unrestricted use of meters in research studies may have blunted the conclusions with regard to the benefits of these devices.

Certain information on a severe asthmatic is required before one can begin to draw up a self-management plan for his or her condition.

The check-list culled from responses to this question by members of Doctors' Reading Club is shown below:

- attacks – frequency, duration, provoking factors, hospitalization
- symptoms – correlation with peak-flow readings
- occupation – restriction of activities
- provoking factors
- for children – height and weight and percentile ratings
- peak flow – ability to use a meter, expected reading, best and worst readings
- current use of medications for asthma – reliever or preventer(s)
- other medical conditions.

4   Peak-flow meters may help patients and doctors to identify the following problems:
- anxiety masquerading as asthma
- fixed airflow obstruction that does not respond to bronchodilators or steroids
- refusal to acknowledge that airflow obstruction exists and may be treatable
- situational asthma, e.g nocturnal, or after exercise or exposure to dust or cold
- asthma requiring prompt treatment.

Several members therefore felt that any asthmatic who requires bronchodilators more than once or twice a week should have a peak-flow meter available until they have developed an understanding of how the condition affects them. Experimenting with the peak-flow meter is likely to help the patient to learn how severe the asthma is and what factors aggravate and relieve it.

5   Members of Doctors' Reading Club suggested that asthmatics or parents of asthmatics should use their peak-flow meters to define their personal best peak flow and their circadian variation, and to define trigger levels that justify intensifying their treatment or consulting their doctor. In particular, a fall in peak flow may precede the onset of symptoms and justify use of inhaled steroids. Short-term loan of a peak-flow meter may be useful for determining whether a patient with a chronic cough or other relevant symptoms is suffering from bronchoconstriction and is benefiting from a therapy. Patients can also use meters to check their responsiveness to steroids and cromoglycate. Trigger factors for asthma can be identified objectively. Two members

wrote that they had devised a printed sheet which they give to patients along with the prescription for the peak-flow meter, advising them on its use.

6 According to these authors good results were achieved with the following policy. Double the dose of inhaled steroid for 2 weeks if the peak-flow rate drops below 85% of personal best. Use a 2-week course of oral steroids if the peak-flow rate drops below 70% of personal best.

7 Use a vacuum cleaner regularly to reduce the content of house-dust mite droppings. Apply a material such as Actomite to eradicate house-dust mites.
Avoid gas appliances, which are associated with high levels of nitrogen dioxide.
Use wood- or coal-burning fires rather than central heating, as these are associated with lower levels of bronchial hyper-reactivity.

8 They harbour four times as much house-dust mite allergen.

9 A high intake of fruit and vegetables, magnesium, vitamin C, selenium and anti-oxidant vitamins, and a low intake of sodium.

10 It reduces static, so fewer particles adhere to the surface of the device.

11 False.

12 False.

13 Ideally one would provide written and verbal instructions covering the following.
   • Use prophylactic drug(s) regularly.
   • Use the nebulizer to give a weight-related dose, e.g. 50–150 mcg salbutamol/kg.
   • Monitor the effect with a paediatric peak-flow meter.
   • Call the doctor, e.g. if the peak flow is less than 60% of that expected for the height of the child 1 h after using one dose from the nebulizer.

14 Patients who use pressurized aerosol canisters of asthma medicines are advised to shake them before use to ensure that the drug and propellant are evenly mixed. If this is done there is no reason to suppose that an inhalation from a near-empty canister will contain less medication than an inhalation from a full one. The fluid in the canister can be heard when one shakes it, and many patients are able to tell when their canisters are nearly empty. Thus the advice to test whether the canister is empty by seeing whether it floats, as suggested in the *BMJ* article, seems to be redundant. Floating is in any case a matter of degree, as the canisters float progressively higher as they empty. The newer inhaler devices provide a means of determining how many puffs of medication are left, and this is of great value, as patients are frequently taken unawares when their canister becomes empty.

15 Asthmatics tend to find that their inhalers are empty at the times when they need them most. Therefore members suggested demonstrating to patients inhalers that are full, half full and nearly empty, and showing them the shake test. They also suggested ensuring that these patients are familiar with the procedure for repeat prescribing. Asthmatics who require frequent treatment should always have a reserve inhaler. Those who have recurring asthmatic crises need to use their peak-flow meters more

frequently in order to be forewarned when their airway condition is deteriorating. The problem will be improved when manufacturers produce transparent canisters or puff counters.

16 He should increase his dose. If any tablets are vomited, they should be replaced. See a doctor at the first hint of feeling unwell.

17 Double the dose at the first warning of smog. Consider a midday dose, as pollution is worst in the afternoon. Avoid strenuous outdoor exercise during periods of pollution. Consider using a car or public transport rather than walking or cycling. Take an indoor swim in hot weather. Cover the face with a mask when outdoors. Drive a car with an air filter.

18 Even when they know that they are being monitored, mothers may not provide their asthmatic toddlers with sufficient doses of bronchodilator and prophylactic medicine to prevent cough and wheeze. Members of Doctors' Reading Club suggested that we address this problem in the following ways.

- Make sure that mothers are aware of the uses of the different types of inhaler, their duration of action, their excellent safety record, and the fact that they are not addictive.
- Provide an instruction leaflet.
- Make more use of long-acting preparations such as salmeterol and steroid inhalers, rather than salbutamol and cromoglycate. Also make more use of inhalers containing a combination of ipratropium and salbutamol, which are more effective than either of these drugs on its own.
- Provide two or more of each type of inhaler so that they can be kept available in convenient places.
- Encourage toddlers to ask their parents for the inhaler when they feel wheezy or 'tight' or have a cough.
- Encourage the use of a monitoring notebook and a peak-flow meter to aid recognition of the problem.
- Advise mothers on measures to eliminate house-dust mite and other irritants.

19 What guideline should we give parents of asthmatics on using prophylactic drugs? If these children are unable to measure peak flow, we have to base the use of prophylactics on frequency of symptoms and use of bronchodilators. There is evidence that prophylactics are underused, leading to impaired health and growth, so it seems wise to err on the generous side in our guideline.

The initial suggestion was that symptoms or use of bronchodilators more often than three times per week justify increased use of prophylaxis. Members commented that this is difficult to understand, and suggested that once weekly was sufficient to justify increased use of prophylactics, particularly as much childhood asthma goes unobserved by parents. If use of bronchodilators is used to indicate a need for increased prophylaxis, there is a danger that parents may use them together and omit to use the prophylactic at other times.

A more comprehensive guideline is needed. Perhaps it should read something like this. 'If your child develops a cold or has recurrent mild cough or wheeze, or has a single prolonged or severe episode of cough or wheeze, increase your use of inhaled steroid and increase it again if the problem does not go away. Continue using the steroid at the increased dose for a further 2 weeks, and then reduce it gradually over the next 3 to 6 weeks, provided that the problem does not return.'

Parents of children using cromoglycate, which is best used at a fixed dose, may be best advised to continue the treatment for 2 to 3 months after the last observed symptoms of asthma, and to reintroduce it at the start of a season when a return of the asthma can be expected.

20 Obviously the condition needs to be of a severity and frequency that justifies oral steroids before a stock of treatment is provided. Members of Doctors' Reading Club also suggested that the patient or carer should have good insight into the condition and know how to monitor and treat it.

21 Possible reasons are that asthmatics with poor mental health have relatively poor compliance, and are less likely to seek medical advice for their asthma.

22 a For the baby with a nocturnal cough, members of Doctors' Reading Club suggested some basic advice to parents on how to minimize or prevent the problem. This included avoiding allergens, particularly house-dust mite, keeping the room as free of dust as possible, and discouraging parental smoking. The risk of asphyxia can be reduced by laying the baby on her back with the head of the cot slightly raised. Airways are less irritable in a warm moist atmosphere, and this can be produced by boiling a kettle or by having a towel soaked in boiling water by the radiator at night. Members' views on drug treatment of a baby with nocturnal cough were very varied, reflecting the lack of consensus in the literature. Beta-two-receptors are commonly believed not to develop until the second or third year of life, so several members suggested ipratropium or oxitropium aerosol rather than salbutamol as their first-line treatment, delivered via a coffee-cup mask – which is less frightening than a large plastic spacer and has the further advantage of not having a valve which the baby might be too weak to open on inspiration. If the nocturnal cough is prolonged for more than 1 week, several members suggested adding an inhaled steroid or a small dose of theophylline syrup.

b There was less controversy about treating the 7-year-old who experiences pro-longed coughing every time he catches a cold. Most members opted for a steroid aerosol at the onset of the cold, supplemented with a bronchodilator aerosol once cough and wheeze start. The steroid needs to be continued until symptoms have resolved and the peak flow has returned to normal levels for 1 week, and its use should then be tapered in accordance with peak-flow observations.

c The 65-year-old man with prolonged wheeze is at particular risk of death due to hypoxia provoking arrhythmia. The response to nebulized salbutamol and beclomethasone may be short-lived and symptoms may return at night, when there is reluctance to summon (or provide) medical assistance. A peak-flow rate of 220 L/min is less than 50% of that expected for a 65-year-old of medium height, and a pulse rate of 95 beats/min and respiration rate of 18 breaths/min suggest that hypoxia is persisting. Members were divided as to how to monitor the patient after his response to initial treatment. Much would depend on the patient's (and his wife's) understanding of the dangers, and their ability to check the peak-flow rate hourly and respond to a recurrence of the symptoms. However, few hospital doctors would quibble about admitting such a patient for oxygen, steroid and bronchodilator treatment and observation.

Medical treatment

1 a False – it should be introduced at a high dose in order to abort an episode, and then reduced gradually as the condition permits.

b True – if low-dose inhaled steroids are insufficient.

c False – cromoglycate and inhaled steroids are equally favoured.

2 a False.

b True.

c True.

3 40 mg oral prednisolone.

4 Prednisolone 1 mg/kg twice daily for 3–4 days. Such courses provided up to six times per year will not have a significant effect on the child's growth.

5 False.

6 True.

7 True – a 16–50% reduction was shown in the growth of the lower leg during treatment of children aged 6–13 years with doses of budesonide between 200 and 800 mcg/day for 18 days.

8 a True – but at only 90 mL the increase in FEV_1 compared to the recordings in the placebo group was of minor clinical significance.

b True – perhaps the dry-powder inhaler acts as an irritant, as a similar increase was noted in the placebo group.

c False – little difference was found between the placebo and the treatment groups in frequency or severity of infections, although the total duration of symptoms was about 35% lower in the patients on beclomethasone.

9 a True.

b True.

c True.

d True.

10 Intal and Atrovent or Oxivent inhalers fit the Nebuhaler but not the Volumatic.

11 True.

12 False.

13 **a** True.

    b True.

    c True.

    d True.

    e True.

14 **a** Salmeterol has not been trialled in this use, but it does appear to be a rational choice.

    b The combination of inhaled salbutamol and inhaled steroid is the usual choice of most doctors.

    c It is unwise to stop salbutamol while asthma symptoms continue.

    d A combination of salbutamol and cromoglycate is a poor choice for nocturnal asthma in an adult.

15 Reflux of gastric acid causing oesophageal irritation may provoke a vagal reflex, causing bronchoconstriction.

16 PACT data can be used to show the ratio of prescriptions for bronchodilators to prescriptions for asthma prophylactic drugs.

17 They should be administered in this way to reduce the ratio of steroid deposited on the oropharynx to steroid deposited in the lungs.

18 Increase the dose greatly during an acute attack and reduce it gradually thereafter. Ten puffs of salbutamol delivered via a spacer tube are as effective as a nebule delivered by nebulizer.

19 Small babies, especially those with acute asthma, may be unable to open the valve on inspiration.

20 Methotrexate theophylline and montelukast to control asthma, and HRT or biphosphonates for osteoporosis. If the patient is not already using inhaled steroids, attempt to substitute them for part of the dose of oral prednisolone.

21 **a** False – trials have yielded conflicting results, and no acaricides are completely free from toxicity. Air filters and ionizers have not been shown to be effective either, although air filters on vacuum cleaners are probably advantageous.

    b True – its long duration of action makes it suitable for controlling nocturnal asthma or frequent exercise-induced asthma, but these conditions also benefit from use of a prophylactic steroid.

    c False – if cromoglycate does not provide adequate control it is better to withdraw it and substitute an inhaled steroid.

    d True.

    e True – 30 L/min compared to 90 L/min.

22 Suggest that the patient monitors peak flow regularly during the first 2 weeks of treatment.

23 False.

24 **a** Metered-dose inhaler – patient with poor technique: 7–13%.
    b Metered-dose inhaler – patient with good technique: 13–19%.
    c Metered-dose inhaler with spacer chamber: 16–21%.
    d Dry-powder inhaler – fast inhalation: 22–32%.
    e Dry-powder inhaler – slow inhalation: 15%.

25 Record peak flow twice daily while taking prednisolone 30 mg or 40 mg once daily in the morning for 10–14 days.

26 This study found a requirement for treatment for 4 h in the treated group, compared to 11.5 h in the control group.

27 44%.

28 Acute angle-closure glaucoma.

29 **a** True.
    b True.

BLOOD PRESSURE

Assessment

1 What happens to a young man's blood pressure when it is recorded by a young woman?

BMJ. **316**: 562

2 Detection.

a What are the 5-year inception rates for hypertension estimated for men and women in this adult population in a mining village?

b In 1991, roughly what proportion of young male adult Londoners had their blood pressure recorded on their GP notes?

BMJ. **306**: 431–2

3 When seeing a newly diagnosed hypertensive:

a How may the results of a full blood count influence management? (*2 points*)

b How may ECG findings influence management? (*2 points*)

c Why should one be cautious about prescribing an ACE inhibitor to someone with peripheral vascular disease?

BMJ. **306**: 983–7

4 Slimmer people have lower blood pressure. What methodological problem might lead one to doubt this assertion?

BMJ. **302**: 1604–5

5 Blood pressure. (*True/False*)

a Ambulatory recordings predict reduction in LV mass by drug treatment better than do measurements of clinic blood pressure.

b Patients whose blood pressures dip at night are very unlikely to have sec-ondary hypertension.

c Patients whose blood pressures do not dip at night are likely to have sec-ondary hypertension.

d About half of all hypertensive people have white-coat hypertension.

e White-coat hypertension attenuates with repeated observations.

f The British Society for Hypertension recommends use of a 13 × 35 cm cuff for adults with circumference up to 42 cm when performing ambula-tory monitoring.

g The cuff should be applied to the non-dominant arm for ambulatory moni-toring.

h Diastolic blood pressure between 90 and 100 mmHg justifies treatment if there is left ventricular hypertrophy in a middle-aged person.

i Symptoms of phaeochromocytoma include headache.

j Two digital electronic sphygmomanometers have been approved for home recording of blood pressure.

BMJ. **313**: 1535–40 (review article)

---

6 Ambulatory monitoring.

a If ambulatory monitoring of blood pressure is used, what cut-off point for daytime systolic and diastolic blood pressure currently seems to be appropriate for selecting patients for treatment with an antihypertensive?

b What advantages does ambulatory monitoring of blood pressure have over measuring it in the surgery?

BMJ. **305**: 716–17, 1062–6

Br J Gen Pract. **42**: 402–3

---

7 Blood-pressure readings obtained with an automatic inflation monitor during sleep are likely to be falsely high. (*True/False*)

BMJ. **308**: 820–3

---

8 What clinical or laboratory observations suggest a need for early treatment in borderline hypertension? (*4 points*)

BMJ. **307**: 1541–6

---

9 Patients with renovascular hypertension usually have less diurnal variation in blood pressure than do those with primary hypertension. (*True/False*)

BMJ. **308**: 630–2

10 Negroid people with hypertension: (*True/False*)

  a have a worse prognosis than whites

  b respond better than whites to ACE inhibitors

  c are more prone to left ventricular hypertrophy than are white hypertensives.

  BMJ. **308**: 1011–14

Management

1 The following nutrients have been reported to reduce blood pressure: (*True/False*)

  a garlic

  b fish oil.

  Br J Gen Pract. **46**: 187–90

2 The blood pressures of patients with borderline hypertension will drop if they avoid coffee. (*True/False*)

  BMJ. **303**: 1235–7

3 How many poorly controlled hypertensives would need to have their systolic blood pressures reduced to below 150/90 mmHg for 5 years in order to prevent one stroke?

  BMJ. **314**: 272–6 (report of case-control study)

4 With regard to treated hypertensive men in their early fifties, what difference in mortality from all causes and from coronary artery disease is to be expected in the next 22 years compared to normotensive men of the same age?

  BMJ. **316**: 167–71 (report of prospective study)

5 According to MRC guidelines on treatment for hypertension, what should be the cut-off points in diastolic blood pressure for treating hypertension in patients aged:

  a under 45 years

  b over 65 years?

  BMJ. **310**: 574

6 The authors of the article referenced below have devised a scheme which enables doctors to base a decision on whether to treat borderline hypertension on an estimate of the probability that the patient will suffer a cardiovascular event in the next 10 years, calculated from an assessment of all of that patient's risk factors. What limitations are there in accepting this approach to deciding whether to offer treatment? (*3 points*)

BMJ. **306**: 107–9

7 The author of the article referenced below concludes that lowering the blood pressure of male hypertensives with left ventricular hypertrophy on their ECGs is likely to increase their risk of myocardial infarction.

  a What mechanism may account for this finding?

  b What misgivings do you have about accepting this conclusion, based on the author's data and his analysis? (*4 points*)

BMJ. **308**: 681–5

8 First-line antihypertensives can be classified as thiazide diuretics, beta-blockers, ACE inhibitors and calcium antagonists. Which class would you choose for each of the following patients, all of whom have a blood pressure averaging 175/110 mmHg, and no evidence of renal damage? State a reason for your choice.

  a A 67-year-old man with nocturia once per night, fatigue after moderate exertion, and LV strain on ECG.

  b A fit 50-year-old man with a normal ECG.

  c A fit 50-year-old woman with a normal ECG.

BMJ. **302**: 352–3

9 What percentage of unselected white patients with diastolic blood pressure of 95–120 mmHg would you expect to achieve a blood pressure of less than 90 mmHg at 8 weeks if they are allocated to treatment with:

  a atenolol

  b hydrochlorothiazide

  c nitrendipine

  d enalapril.

BMJ. **315**: 154–8 (trial report)

10 What class of antihypertensive appeared ineffective in treating hypertension in smokers in the MRC trials? (*1 point*)

BMJ. **306**: 1337

11 The following drug classes have been shown to have an additive antihypertensive effect when used in combination: (*True/False*)

  a diuretic and calcium antagonist

  b ACE inhibitor and calcium antagonist.

BMJ. **307**: 1541–5

12 Renal artery stenosis and ACE inhibitors.

  a What is the reported prevalence of renal artery stenosis in the following groups of patients:

   i those with peripheral vascular disease

   ii those with coronary artery disease

   iii those with type 2 diabetes?

  b What is the limitation of using a rise in serum creatinine after several days of use of ACE inhibitors as a screening method for damage due to the combination with renal artery stenosis?

  c What alternative methods seem practicable to screen for renal artery stenosis?

BMJ. **316**: 1921 (editorial)

13 A hypertensive patient taking atenolol who develops intermittent claudication should have nifedipine substituted for the atenolol. (*True/False*)

BMJ. **303**: 1100–4

14 There is scant evidence from clinical trials that patients over the age of 80 years benefit from taking antihypertensives, so the authors of this article recommend that when patients taking antihypertensives reach the age of 80 years they should have a trial of withdrawal of treatment. Do you agree with this? State two reasons for your point of view.

BMJ. **304**: 412–16

15 When managing hypertension in the elderly: (*True/False*)

  a isolated systolic high blood pressure does not require treatment

  b blood pressure readings immediately after a stroke are representative of the long-term blood pressure.

BMJ. **305**: 750–2

16 What physiological reason may underlie the finding in this study that metoprolol was a more effective antihypertensive than isradipine (a calcium antagonist) for obese hypertensives, while the reverse was true for slim sub-jects? (*2 points*)

What reservations do you have about accepting the principle that beta-blockers are better for obese hypertensives and calcium antagonists for slim ones?

BMJ. **307**: 537–40

17 Patients whose hypertension is well controlled on nifedipine without any symptomatic side-effects should have an alternative drug substituted. Do you agree? Give your reasons. (*2 or more points*)

BMJ. **312**: 1143–5 (review)

18 Which of your hypertensive patients currently on therapy might you consider for a trial of withdrawal of therapy?

BMJ. **303**: 324–5, 643–5

ANSWERS

Assessment

1   In this study the systolic blood pressure of young men was about 5 mmHg higher when measured by young women than when measured in other conditions.

2   a   26/1000 for men and 18/1000 for women.

    b   10–30%.

3   a   Macrocytosis suggests that alcohol is a contributory factor.
Polycythaemia is a separate risk factor.

    b   The presence of ischaemia suggests that a beta-blocker would be particularly beneficial.
The presence of left ventricular hypertrophy suggests that treatment is indicated at a lower cut-off point than usual.

    c   Peripheral vascular disease is associated with a 40% prevalence of renal artery stenosis, which is a contraindication to the use of an ACE inhibitor.

4   Unless cuff sizes are finely graded, more pressure will be required to occlude the brachial artery in an obese arm than in a thin one.

5   a   True.

    b   True.

    c   False.

    d   False (correct proportion is 10–20%).

    e   False – patients whose blood pressure falls with repeated clinic observations are termed white-coat responders.

    f   True.

    g   True.

    h   True.

    i   True.

    j   True – The Omron HEP75CP (Tel 01273 495033) and the Takeda UA-751 (Fax: 00 3 5391 6148).

6   a   Authors variously suggest 160/95 mmHg and 91 mmHg diastolic.

    b   It avoids white-coat hypertension, found in about 22–30% of patients.
It avoids observer bias and digit preference.
A representative reading is obtained in 1 day, so the patient is less likely to be lost to follow-up.
More readings are taken so a more precise estimate is obtained.
There is a better correlation of blood pressure with end-organ damage.

7 True – inflation of the cuff alarms the patient.

8 Left ventricular hypertrophy on the ECG or echocardiogram, the presence of other risk factors or of proteinuria or a raised creatinine or urea concentration.

9 True.

10 a True.
   b False – they also respond less well to beta-blockers.
   c True.

Management

1 a True.
  b True.

2 False.

3 86.

4 A total mortality of 38% is expected in the treated hypertensive men, compared to 29% in the normotensive men. A mortality of 22% from coronary artery disease is expected in the treated hypertensives, compared to 11% in the normotensive men.

5 a 100 mmHg.
  b 90 mmHg.

6 The idea of incorporating other risk factors in the assessment seems sound, but members identified the following flaws in the detail.

   The decision aid would exclude from treatment many younger hypertensives who might derive a considerable increase in longevity as a result of treatment, although this would be achieved at a much greater prescribing cost. An analysis based on added life years might be more useful than one based on expected time to death.

   The decision aid made no use of information on the patient's exercise or diet habits. Coronary risk factors change with life-style, and those who adopt this approach need to determine how much time and effort is worth expending before invoking the decision aid.

   The relative importance of hypertension as a risk factor is greater at higher blood pressures, but the proposed scheme does not make allowance for this. It might be difficult to dissuade a doctor from treating a middle-aged patient with a blood pressure consistently around 170/105 mmHg just because he had no other risk factors.

   Finally, the authors chose an arbitrary figure of 20% risk of cardiovascular disease in 10 years as the determinant that justifies use of antihypertensives. The choice of figure might best be discussed with the patient or (not so satisfactory) chosen by consensus of a representative panel.

7 The author of the original article found that the risk of myocardial infarct increased, although not significantly, with diastolic blood pressure in males 1 year after initiation

of antihypertensive treatment if the patients had normal electrocardiograms, whereas it fell significantly with increasing diastolic blood pressure if the ECG suggested ischaemia or hypertrophy, or both. Overall, the risk of myocardial infarction fell with increasing diastolic blood pressure after initiation of treatment. No similar relationship was found for women or for systolic blood pressure. The implication is that if a hypertensive man's ECG shows LVH and his diastolic blood pressure falls considerably in response to antihypertensive treatment, his risk of infarct is increased, possibly because treatment has reduced his myocardial blood flow.

There have been previous reports of a J-curve linking risk of myocardial infarct to diastolic blood pressure, but this is the first time that LVH or ischaemia on the ECG have been suggested to predict those individuals who may be put at risk by use of antihypertensive drugs. GPs discussing this question felt the story would have been more convincing if the data from women had shown a similar trend, and if more than one blood pressure reading had been incorporated in the analysis.

The gender difference is not easily explained, and puts a question mark over the hypothesis. Death certificates were used as one method of identifying myocardial infarcts, but are suspect for this purpose.

The antihypertensives used in the study were propranolol or metoprolol and a thiazide, either singly or in combination. An interaction seems likely between the choice of antihypertensive and the influence of LVH on mortality, but this was not discussed by the author. The study made no mention of overall mortality, and the risk of stroke would almost certainly be reduced by lowering the blood pressure, even in those with LVH. Alcohol causing cardiomyopathy may be a confounding factor. A prospective trial may be needed for a definitive answer.

8 GPs discussing this question mentioned the following considerations.

- In favour of diuretics are their low cost and beneficial effects in congestive cardiac failure, but impotence and the slight effects on lipids may be problems. Diuretics also promote retention of calcium, thus possibly reducing osteoporosis, and this factor may favour their use in women in particular.

- In favour of beta-blockers are their relatively low cost and evidence of cardioprotection after myocardial infarction, but cold legs, bronchospasm, tiredness and impotence may be problems. This last problem may make them more suitable for the fit 50-year-old woman than for the man.

- In favour of calcium antagonists there is evidence of protection against episodic vasospasm, and lack of an effect on impotence, but some drugs in this class lower cardiac output, and none have a proven ability to reduce cardiac mortality. Some older formulations do not confer a 24-hour reduction in blood pressure. They may be the drug of first choice for a man to whom potency is a concern.

- In favour of ACE inhibitors there is a beneficial effect in congestive cardiac failure, possibly favourable metabolic effects, as well as probable renal protection in patients with microalbuminuria, but at a risk of aggravating renal artery stenosis, and the relatively high costs of these drugs have not yet been justified in studies of long-term mortality and morbidity.

9 a 64%.

   b 45%.

   c 45%.

   d 35%.

10 Beta-blockers.

11 a False.

    b True.

12 a i   40%.

     ii 20%.

     iii 10%.

    b The creatinine level will only rise if the renal artery stenosis is bilateral.

    c Duplex scanning with ultrasound. Colour Doppler ultrasound.

13 False – there is no evidence of benefit from the change.

14 GPs discussing this question reached the following conclusions.

    Doctrinaire use of 80 years as a cut-off point is inappropriate. However, in an elderly treated hypertensive patient, quality of life may be more important than long-term protective effect of antihypertensives, so:

- weigh up the discomforts associated with treatment and the effect of having to take treatment on the patient's self-image
- weigh up whether the patient may be precipitated into fatigue, heart failure or arrhythmia if antihypertensives are reduced or stopped
- consider using chest X-ray and/or echocardiography for assessment.

15 a False.

    b False.

16 Obese patients have higher sympathetic activity and lower peripheral resistance. GPs discussing the report reached the following conclusions.

- The report was of a small, short-term trial, limited to white men.
- The trial involved only one drug from each class, so it may not be a class effect.
- Beta-blockers carry more risk of fatigue, airway obstruction and increased lipid levels for obese patients.

17 A large case-control study in America has shown a 58–70% greater risk of myocardial infarction with calcium-channel blockers than with diuretic treatment for hypertension. The increased risk is dose related, whereas for beta-blockers the risk of myocardial infarction decreases with increased dose. A meta-analysis of clinical trials also found a dose-related excess mortality associated with short-acting nifedipine. Possible mechanisms for the bad news about nifedipine are catecholamine surges associated with varying levels of nifedipine linked with reflex tachycardia.

    Members were divided as to whether this would cause them to switch patients on nifedipine to another antihypertensive. Most could see advantages in switching to the longest-acting preparation available, or using it in conjunction with a beta-blocker to inhibit the reflex tachycardia. Others thought that if patients were symptom free and their hypertension was well controlled this information should be weighed against the evidence against nifedipine.

18 Members agreed that the following factors could justify a trial of withdrawing antihypertensive treatment:

- no evidence of organ damage, in particular no LVH on ECG
- only one drug required for control
- numerous recent blood pressure readings were all under 160/90 mmHg
- suffering no intercurrent stress
- a reduction in stress since the time when the diagnosis was made
- a reduction in weight since the time when the diagnosis was made
- lower alcohol consumption if this had previously been high
- feeling dizzy or suffering other side-effects while on treatment
- original readings having been made with a cuff that was too small
- normal blood lipids and a non-smoker.

Three or more blood pressure readings are needed in the weeks after drugs are withdrawn, and a further reading 6 to 12 months thereafter.

CANCER

Aetiology

1 What is the estimated odds ratio for stomach cancer in patients with helico-bacter antibodies?

BMJ. **315**: 1199–201 (research report)

2 What previous occupations might be relevant to the aetiology of primary tumours at the following sites?

a liver.

b urothelium.

c lung.

d nose.

e larynx.

f leukaemia.

g skin.

BMJ. **313**: 615–19 (review article)

3 What form of cancer has been found to be particularly common in garage mechanics, and what may account for this?

BMJ. **311**: 1110 (citation)

Diagnosis and assessment

1 It is reasonable to allow a mouth ulcer to persist for up to 2 months before referring the problem to an oral surgeon. (*True/False*)

BMJ. **308**: 669–70

2 CA125 glycoprotein as a marker for cancer of the ovary or Fallopian tube: (*True/False*)

a is useful for monitoring and surveillance of most cases of ovarian cancer

b is useful for screening premenopausal women.

BMJ. **313**: 1355–8 (research report)

3 In multiple myeloma, why is serum gammaglobulin electrophoresis on its own inadequate as a screening test?

BMJ. **309**: 1033–6

4 With regard to prevention of colonic cancer:

a the finding of a villous adenoma on sigmoidoscopy justifies what further investigation?

b what items of family history justify particular vigilance?

BMJ. **305**: 246–9

5 What clinical features help to differentiate lipomas from sarcomas?

BMJ. **316**: 93–4 (leading article)

6 List the practice policies that are likely to reduce the interval between onset and diagnosis of common cancers.

BMJ. **305**: 419–22

Management

1 You receive an X-ray report showing an almost certain lung tumour in an elderly male patient.

a What further information about the patient will help you to decide whether and how to break the news?

b What information may it be important for the patient to know? (*5 points*)

BMJ. **307**:1502–3

2 A patient with advanced cancer is being cared for by his wife. In addition to his occasional chemotherapy and radiotherapy and symptom relief, what other areas will you seek to cover in a discussion with him and his wife during a home visit? (*4 points*)

BMJ. **306**: 249–50

3 The following will help to maximize quality of life for cancer patients: (*True/False*)

a an exact estimate of life expectancy

b avoiding use of chemotherapy with unpleasant side-effects unless there is a 30% chance of significant benefit

c providing regular access to a senior doctor to discuss treatment policy

d encouraging patients to take up the offer of a counselling service.

BMJ. **305**: 466–9

4 This trial showed positive benefit for women diagnosed as having breast cancer who received about six sessions of cognitive and behavioural therapy. On what topics would such therapy centre?

BMJ. **304**: 675–9

5 **a** What benefits are there for cancer patients in attending meetings of an expressive supportive group?

b How may they find out about a local group?

BMJ. **315**: 812 (letter)

6 The benefits of patient-run self-help groups for cancer victims are well proven. (*True/False*)

BMJ. **316**: 781 (letter)

7 Homecare.

a It is often difficult to arrange adequate homecare for a disabled patient who cannot use the toilet unaided. What medical measures and appliances can help to alleviate the problem?

b What organization can advise cancer sufferers on how to obtain a grant to pay fuel bills or for installation of special equipment?

BMJ. **316**: 373–6 (review)

8 What treatment might you give a patient who has developed a phobia of chemotherapy for cancer, and who thus experiences the side-effects particularly severely?

BMJ. **309**: 1649–53 (review)

9 In cancer palliation, what adjuvants to morphine may be useful for pain due to the following causes?

a Bone metastases.

b Raised intracranial pressure.

c Hepatomegaly.

d Soft tissue infiltration.

e Nerve infiltration.

f Tenesmus or rectal spasm.

BMJ. **315**: 801–4, 867–9(review)

10 Oral corticosteroids in advanced cancer. (*True/False*)

a Prednisolone need only be taken once daily.

b The effect on anorexia may wear off after a few weeks.

c The dose required to initiate improvement may be more than the dose required to maintain it thereafter.

d These drugs may cause prolonged remission of a prostate cancer.

BMJ. **305**: 969–70, 999

11 Treatment of cachexia in cancer patients.

a What benefits and what duration of benefit would you expect from prednisolone 40 mg/day? (*3 points*)

b What benefits would you expect from megestrol acetate 480 mg/day?

c Which symptoms might respond to a prokinetic agent?

BMJ. **315**:1219–22 (review article)

12 Bone metastases. (*True/False*)

a These are found in about one in four women undergoing surgery for breast cancer.

b External beam radiotherapy provides immediate relief from the resulting pain.

c Introducing oestrogenic treatment provides only slight relief from pain due to metastatic prostatic cancer.

BMJ. **303**: 429–30

13 What benefits have been demonstrated in clinical trials for the long-term prescription of oral biphosphonates in patients with myeloma and metastatic breast cancer?

BMJ. **309**:1233 (letter)

14 Why do many patients with myeloma benefit from a high fluid intake?

BMJ. **309**: 1033–6

15 Emergencies in cancer care.

a What clinical features suggest hypercalcaemia?

b How do you correct serum calcium for the albumen concentration?

c What is the emergency treatment for severe hypercalcaemia?

d What clinical features suggest obstruction of the superior vena cava?

e What is the emergency treatment for obstruction of the superior vena cava?

f A 65-year-old man with a history of cancer has noted mild girdle pain around his chest, which is worse on coughing, for the past 3 days. Why is it important to question and examine him carefully for other neurological signs and ensure that he comes back for follow-up?

g What is the first investigation of choice for suspected cord compression? (*1 point*)

BMJ. **315**:1525–8 (review)

ANSWERS

Aetiology

1 The odds ratio for stomach cancer in patients with helicobacter antibodies has been estimated to be four.

2 a PVC production.

   b Work in a chemical plant, laboratory, aluminium works, gas or coking plant, paint shop or dyeworks.

   c Exposure to asbestos in asbestos production, building industry, vehicle-building, dockyard, navy, or exposure to coal tars in the coke industry.

   d Boot- and shoe-making, cabinet-making, manufacture of isopropyl alcohol.

   e Soap-making or chemical works involving exposure to sulphuric acid fumes.

   f Petrol industry, boot and shoe manufacture, exposure to ethylene oxide in medical sterilization.

   g Exposure to mineral oil in engineering, exposure to soot in chimney cleaning, exposure to coal tars in the gas and coke industries.

3 Leukaemia and lymphatic neoplasms, which are attributed to washing the hands with petrol, which contains benzene.

Diagnosis and assessment

1 False – a maximum of 3 weeks is suggested.

2 a True – it is raised in 85% of epithelial ovarian cancer.

   b False – the low incidence of ovarian cancer in premenopausal women and the prevalence of other conditions associated with a raised level of CA125 limit its use until after the menopause.

3 a 20% of cases have myeloma protein in the urine but no paraprotein band in the serum.

4 a Colonoscopy.

   b Colon carcinoma, adenomatous polyposis, carcinoma of the ovary, breast or uterus.

5 Soft tissue sarcomas become more common with increasing age, and are usually larger than lipomas at presentation – typically around 9 cm. They usually present with no pain or loss of function. They may be tethered to the muscles, and may be growing

rapidly. Open biopsy may be inconclusive, as unrepresentative tissue may be sampled and pathologists may lack experience.

6 Diagnosing cancers at a stage when they are treatable is an important goal for general practice. GPs discussing this question came up with a varied selection of practical points to achieve this objective. They can be divided into screening exercises, health education (so that patients will bring relevant symptoms to medical attention early) and good practice (so that suspect findings will be investigated promptly).

With regard to the suggestions on screening, cervical smears and mammograms are accepted routines. In addition, the urine dipsticks used for people over 50 years of age should include a test for red cells. Prostate-specific antigen is looking increasingly useful for the early detection of prostate cancer, and should be added to the request list when blood from elderly men is sent for biochemistry analysis. Faecal occult blood samples are messy to collect, requiring defaecation into a dry container, but middle-aged and elderly people with a family history of bowel cancer should perhaps be providing such samples annually.

GPs' suggestions on health education might usefully be put into practice leaflets. Mention could be made of the value of the cervical smear for women, and of self-examination for testicular cancer in young men. Breast self-examination could be taught to women over 35 years of age when they come for their cervical smears or family planning appointments.

Patients could be advised to let the doctor know early on if they note altered bowel habit or blood in the stools or urine.

One doctor mentioned that if patients are to bring their worrying symptoms to medical attention, the doctor needs to be accessible, tactful and pleasant. He or she will need a high index of suspicion, particularly for digestive symptoms in middle-aged patients, and should be willing to refer for endoscopy rather than rely on antacids or acid-suppressing treatment. He will also need the time to examine patients with suspect symptoms. For those patients in whom a cancer is palpable or highly likely, a telephone call to the hospital unit rather than a routine referral letter will speed up investigation.

Several doctors suggested that practices might audit their recent cases of cancer to determine whether and how they might have been diagnosed earlier.

Management

1 What information is needed about the elderly gentleman whose chest X-ray shows an inoperable tumour before deciding how to break the news to him? First of all, a discussion with a chest physician and knowledge of the patient's symptoms and his general health may be needed to help one gauge the prognosis and the potential benefits of further treatment. Information on the patient's education and occupational background, his psychiatric history, use of medical and recreational drugs and the reason for performing the X-ray might be found in the notes. If he is going to have

to cope with shocking news it would be desirable that he be accompanied home and be with his relatives for the next few days. Asking how he has coped with previous illnesses or with illnesses in relatives may reveal how much of a realist or stoic he is. One may ask him directly if he likes to be kept fully informed or if he prefers to leave things to the experts. A non-specific description such as 'shadow on the lung' may be a suitable way to introduce the X-ray report.

It may comfort the patient to know that he has probably had the shadow for years. Reassurance that you are always available to tell him anything he wants or needs to know may be better than presenting the implications at the first interview. He may also be advised to let you know if he has symptoms, as you can certainly keep them under control. One doctor uses the statement 'I think you and I are going to be seeing a lot of each other' to suggest that it is a serious problem, but that the doctor is readily available for help and support.

Several members suggested discussing the problem with relatives. However, if the patient is free of dementia it may cause considerable tension in the household if relatives are well informed of the prognosis and the patient is not.

When the patient is more fully aware of the implications of the X-ray report, he may need to be reassured that there is no mistake in the report or the prognosis, but that all possible steps will be taken to keep him comfortable. One may ask about occupational exposure to asbestos or other dusts with a view to ascertaining whether there is a possibility of a claim for compensation. It may be relevant to advise the family about claiming Disabled Living Allowance under the special rules, and to tell them about local facilities for home nursing and hospice care.

2 • The carer's welfare, anxieties, and support network.
   • The quality of communication between the patient and his wife, and the degree to which they share an understanding of the diagnosis.
   • Attitudes to respite care and help from a hospice.
   • Practical aids in the home, e.g. commode, wheelchair, etc.
   • DSS benefits.
   • Services from district nurses, specialist nurses, social services, cancer charities and religious bodies.

3 a True.
   b False – most patients want chemotherapy even if there is only a slim chance of benefit.
   c True.
   d True.

4 • The meaning of cancer to the individual.
   • Coping strategies.
   • Identifying personal strengths and raising self-esteem.
   • Overcoming feelings of helplessness.
   • Identifying and challenging negative thoughts.
   • Using imagination and role play to cope with impending stressful events.

- Encouraging activities that give a feeling of achievement and pleasure.
- Encouraging the patient's expression of their feelings to their spouse.
- Teaching progressive muscular relaxation.

5 a Potential benefits include improved mood, reduced maladaptive coping responses and reduced pain.

   b Through Cancerlink (17 Britannia Street, London WC1, Tel 0171 833 2451) or BACUP, Social Services, or the Internet.

6 False.

7 a Suppositories or enemas so that bowel actions are predictable.
      Helpful appliances include raised toilet seat, handrails, commode, wheelchair, hoist, and urinal for use in bed.

   b Macmillan Cancer Relief:

Scotland, Wales and Northern Ireland	Tel 0171 867 9492
North of England	Tel 0171 867 9493
Midlands	Tel 0171 867 9490
South and South-West	Tel 0171 867 9491
London and South-East	Tel 0171 867 9496.

8 A benzodiazepine to cover the 48-h period before and during the chemotherapy is suggested. Further suggestions include an anti-emetic and counselling.

9 • Bone pain – NSAID, biphosphonates, radiotherapy, short-acting opiate for incident pain during movement.
   • Raised intracranial pressure – corticosteroid, e.g. dexamethasone 8 mg daily.
   • Hepatomegaly – NSAID, coeliac plexus block.
   • Soft tissue infiltration – NSAID or corticosteroid.
   • Nerve infiltration – antidepressant, e.g. amitriptyline 25–75 mg nocte, anti-convulsant, e.g. sodium valproate in doses up to 1600 mg/day, anti-arrhythmic, e.g mexiletine 50–200 mg tds, transcutaneous nerve stimulation, acupuncture.
   • Tenesmus or rectal spasm – antispasmodic, smooth muscle relaxant.

10 a True.
    b True.
    c True.
    d True.

11 a Steroid treatment such as prednisolone, 40 mg/day, is likely to improve anorexia and weakness, but does not give a significant improvement in caloric intake. The benefit usually only lasts for up to 3–4 weeks.

    b Progestogen treatment such as megestrol acetate, 480 mg/day, is likely to bring about a lasting improvement in appetite, caloric intake, nutritional intake and fatigue, both in cancer cachexia and in AIDS.

    c Nausea and early satiety may respond to prokinetic agents.

12 a True.

    b False – relief may be delayed for up to 2 weeks.

    c False – 60–90% of sufferers obtain relief for a median of 12–20 months.

13 Prevention of bone secondaries, relief of bone pain, lower incidence of hypercalcae-mia, fewer pathological fractures, and less need for palliative radiotherapy.

14 Myeloma protein is deposited in the proximal tubule at low flow rates, causing hypercalcaemia, renal failure and lethargy.

15 a Nausea, vomiting, constipation, dehydration, drowsiness, confusion and cardiac arrhythmia.

    b For every 1 g/L that the serum albumen exceeds 40 g/L, deduct 0.02 mmol/L from the serum calcium. Conversely, for every 1 gm/L that the serum calcium is less than 40 g/L, add 0.02 mmol/L to the serum calcium.

    c Two litres of saline infusion, followed by intravenous biphosphonate. Recheck serum calcium, urea and electrolytes after 3 days and consider maintenance treatment with biphosphonates.

    d Dyspnoea, headache that is worse on stooping, dizziness, visual changes, swelling of the face, neck and arms, peri-orbital oedema, non-pulsatile distended neck veins, suffused conjunctivae, cyanosis, and dilated veins on the upper chest.

    e High-dose steroids, and possibly radiotherapy or stenting.

    f Spinal cord compression presents in many ways, including nerve-root pain, weakness, numbness, and altered bladder and bowel function. Early investigation with an MRI scan and prompt surgical treatment may pre-empt motor paralysis.

    g Magnetic resonance imaging (MRI).

CHRONIC FATIGUE

1 A patient has suffered intermittent fluctuating fatigue affecting mental and bodily functions for more than half the time for more than 6 months. What is the prognosis?

BMJ. **308**: 1297–300

2 According to a DSS report the following are factors that indicate good and poor prognoses for chronic fatigue syndrome. Are there any modifications you might suggest based on your own experience or reading?

Good prognosis:

- a definite history of viral illness
- a pattern of evolution towards recovery
- an early diagnosis aimed at eliminating physical disorders and identifying psychiatric illness and complicating psychosocial factors
- a management regime involving physical, psychological and social elements that concentrate on modifying the patient's life-style, striking a balance between overactivity and the risks of deconditioning, and taking a stepwise approach towards achieving functional improvement while addressing factors such as sleep disturbance.

Poor prognosis:

- onset of symptoms without any clear precipitating factor, but set against a complex background of adverse psychological and social factors or occurring after a severe infective illness
- severe and unremitting symptoms, particularly if lasting for over 4 years, and the presence of multiple symptoms, especially those suggesting somatization
- delayed diagnosis and especially self-diagnosis, with the patient becoming convinced of a single cause to the exclusion of all others
- a management regime that overemphasizes the importance of complete rest or advocates a rapid return to pre-illness levels of physical activity,

and failure to recognize the need to treat such features as depressive illness or sleep disturbance.

BMJ. **313**:885 (letter)

3 What sideroom or laboratory investigations do you feel are justified in a 35-
year-old mother and part-time nurse who gives a 6-month history of dis-
abling physical and mental fatigue as her only abnormality on history and
examination?

Br J Gen Pract. **41**: 339–42

4 What advice on activity do you give to patients with chronic fatigue syndrome?

BMJ. **309**:1515 (letter)

5 'Doctor, I've been feeling terribly tired for 2 months now since I had a dose of
the flu. All I want to do is rest in bed. I know all your blood tests came back
showing nothing abnormal, but can I have a note for school to explain that I
need more time off?' The patient is a 15-year-old schoolgirl of high ability
and stable home circumstances who comes with her mother to see her GP.
Can you think of a list of headings to raise in discussion of the problem?

BMJ. **308**: 732–3, 797

6 What are the potential disadvantages of arranging home tuition for a child
with chronic fatigue syndrome? (*2 or more points*)

BMJ. **314**: 1635–6

7 What sort of exercise programme seems appropriate for someone with
chronic fatigue syndrome?

BMJ. **314**: 1647–51 (research report)

ANSWERS

1 Of the order of 20% of cases recover, 15% show improvement, 40% have a fluctuating course, 15–20% remain severely affected and 5–10% deteriorate.

2 On the basis of their experience, GPs suggested several more prognostic associations, concentrating particularly on motivational aspects.

Good prognosis:

- youth
- intelligence
- objectivity
- good employment record
- good longstanding family relationships
- good record of personal self-care
- improvement in personal circumstances
- shared understanding of the illness and the prognosis with the doctors.

Poor prognosis:

- unsatisfactory work experience and poor employment record
- previous episodes of poorly explained ill health
- poor employment or business prospects
- excessive use of alcohol or recreational drugs
- obesity
- evidence that the sick role provides secondary gain as a refuge from other stresses
- evidence that the sick role is needed in order to maintain stable but unhelpful dynamics in the household
- poor relationships at home
- other members of the household have similar problems
- an obsessive search for physical cures from alternative medicines
- anxiety rather than support from relatives.

3 A comprehensive list derived from suggestions from practising GPs might include urinalysis, full blood count, ESR, CPK, fasting blood glucose, liver function tests, TSH, urea and electrolytes, creatine kinase, protein electrophoresis, monospot, CVP_1 and a chest X-ray.

4 Patients with chronic fatigue syndrome commonly suffer a setback in their recovery, an increase in muscle ache and an increased risk of minor infection if they exceed their limits. Often an increase in activity may be comfortable at the time but can provoke increased fatigue the next day. As one GP who specializes in this area describes it: 'You have to think of the illness as a fire that is out of control. If you exhaust your body it will fan the flames. So be content to live within the limits of activity that are

comfortable at the time and on the next day, and you will starve the illness of oxygen and it will slowly die away.' He therefore advises patients to keep a diary recording their time out of bed, their time on their feet, and the severity of their symptoms on a scale of 0–5 ranging from perfectly well to the worst ever experienced. Exceeding a score of 2 is a sign of overdoing it. Within a few days the patient will have learned the appropriate limits. Patients who have suffered the illness for more than 6 months are advised to stick to these limits for at least 1 month before gradually raising them. Those with shorter-term fatigue states can try increasing their activities more quickly while maintaining their monitoring. Incidentally, SSRIs are acquiring a reputation for improving exercise tolerance in these patients even in the absence of depression, and a small dose of a sedative antidepressant in the evening often helps to restore a normal sleep pattern, which also aids recovery.

5   A teenage girl with persistent fatigue as her only symptom has had several blood tests come back negative. No clues have been found to suggest a physical cause for her problem, but the fatigue remains. Perhaps it would be worth enquiring yet again about myalgia and checking for alteration in weight before explaining that no physical cause can be found for the problem and at present it is not worth pursuing that avenue further.

Members also suggested speaking to the teenager alone, asking for her thoughts on the cause of the problem, and making specific enquiries about other symptoms of depression. Then it would be useful to speak to her and her mother separately about social circumstances or recent events that might be contributing to the problem. In particular it would be worth checking whether the girl has unrealistic ambitions or is making excessive demands of herself, whether she is subject to intimidation at school, and whether she has someone in whom she can readily confide. Has she endured any recent failures or frustrations? Have there been illnesses or bereavements in the family or among friends that are causing her to worry? Are there worries at home about the parental relationship or financial security? Do the girl or her parents abuse coffee, alcohol or leisure drugs?

Under the circumstances most rational teenagers would be worried. Lack of concern would suggest that the girl is masking a poor relationship with adult figures in her life.

Several members suggested a trial of SSRI antidepressants even in the absence of a full-blown picture of clinical depression.

When advising the family, members suggested that the patient should keep a diary of her activities, bedtimes and sleep pattern, and that she should aim to do what schoolwork she could. Sensible habits of sleep, leisure and diet should be discussed. A letter to the school would be useful, and the doctor might explain that no physical cause has been found for the problem and the girl should be encouraged to attend so long as this does not overtire her. Non-attendance at PT and games might be suggested if these activities overtire the girl.

6   Arranging home tuition may aggravate school phobia, increase the child's adoption of the sick role, lead to social isolation, result in the child taking less exercise, and may set a precedent for siblings. Moreover, tutoring at home is troublesome, it is usually done

in the evening when the child is least able to concentrate, and it is difficult to arrange for the whole range of subjects to be covered.

7 This author suggests starting with 5–15 min of exercise per day to 40% of maximum oxygen uptake (approximately 50% of maximal heart rate [200 – age in years] beats/min). Increase this by 1–2 min at weekly intervals until exercising for 30 min. Then increase work output to 60% of maximum oxygen uptake. If fatigue is noted, continue at the same intensity and duration of exercise until the fatigue diminishes.

DERMATOLOGY

Skin treatments – miscellaneous

1 What treatments are available for hyperhidosis? (*5 points*)

BMJ. **306**: 1221

BMJ. **310**: 116

BMJ. **314**: 1562

2 List three or more treatments worthy of consideration for chilblains.

BMJ. **303**: 913–16

3 Calamine lotion is an effective treatment for a painful itchy rash. (*True/False*)

BMJ. **305**: 966

4 What creams and ointments contain peanut oil, which may be dangerous to those who are allergic to peanuts? (*3 points*)

BMJ. **313**: 299 (correspondence)

5 Measuring skin creams.

a What does a fingertip of skin cream weigh? What area of skin will it cover?

b How much suncream will it take to protect the whole body surface to the thickness used when determining the sun protection factor?

BMJ. **313**: 690, 942 (letters)

6 What warning on routine self-care is worth giving to people with skin weakened by prolonged use of oral or topical steroids?

BMJ. **313**: 1024 (citation)

7 What advice might you give patients on how to eliminate fleas from carpets and pets? (*3 points*)

BMJ. **310**: 672

8 Name the household remedy for hyperaesthetic skin.

BMJ. **307**: 273

9 What warning might usefully be given to people applying alcohol-based lotions?

BMJ. **315**: 198 (case report)

10 List treatments for vitiligo that are:

a disease modifying (*4 points*)

b camouflaging (*3 points*)

c protective (*1 point*).

BMJ. **315**: 88 (personal view)

11 Terminal care.

a What oral treatments would you suggest for the following problems in terminal care?

  i A malignant ulcer with a foul smell.

  ii Itch. (*6 points*)

b What topical treatments or dressings would be appropriate for the following?

  i An ulcer with minimal discharge but surrounded by necrotic tissue.

  ii An ulcer with heavy exudate.

  iii Weeping dermatitis on a limb affected by lymphoedema.

BMJ. **315**: 1002–5 (review)

Acne

1 When treating acne: (*True/False*)

a contraceptives containing desogesterol may aggravate the problem

b minocycline appears not to induce bacterial resistance

c oral tetracycline is likely to cause fluorescence under ultraviolet light

d topical clindamycin may cause hyperpigmentation

e intralesional triamcinolone is useful for early scars.

BMJ. **308**: 831–3

2 To prevent the emergence of antibiotic-resistant strains of propionibacteria in acne lesions the following policies are recommended: (*True/False*)

a use of rotational antibiotics

b combined use of an oral and a topical antibiotic

c use of benzoyl peroxide lotions.

BMJ. **306**: 55–6

3 Inhaled steroids can exacerbate acne. (*True/False*)

BMJ. **305**: 1000

4 With which psychiatric problems is isotetinoin associated ?

BMJ. **316**: 723 (news item)

5 What skin disorder may be induced by minocycline?

Br J Gen Pract. **306**: 173

6 What rare serious side-effects seem to be much more common with minocycline than with tetracycline? (*4 points*)

BMJ. **312**: 138 (review)

Skin infections

1 What organisms are most likely to cause skin infections on the chin or cheek in a regular player of a contact sport? (*4 points*)

BMJ. **308**: 1702–6

2 What incidence of post-herpetic neuralgia would you expect in patients aged over 60 years with herpes zoster, based on the results of this study of matched patients:

a if treated with oral acyclovir

b if treated with placebo?

BMJ. **309**: 1124

3 What chemicals make it possible to hook out head lice with a fine-toothed comb? (*2 points*)

BMJ. **314**: 84 (citation)

4 Erythema infectiosum (slapped cheek syndrome due to parvovirus B19). (*True/False*)

a The causative virus can also cause aplastic crises in vulnerable individuals.

b About 90% of adults are seropositive.

c Outbreaks of the disease usually occur in the late summer.

d The arthralgia which affected adults may suffer afterwards is usually most evident in the hands or feet.

e About 30% of pregnancies complicated by the infection in the first two trimesters result in fetal loss.

f The virus is commonly transmitted in blood transfusions.

BMJ. **311**: 1549–51 (review)

Fungal infections

1 What would be the treatment of choice for the following fungal nail infections?

a Dermatophyte infection restricted to the distal and lateral margins of the nail.

b Candida infection restricted to the margin of a nail.

c A severe infection of the whole toenail bed with dermatophytes.

d A severe infection of the whole toenail with a non-dermatophyte mould.

BMJ. **311**: 1277–81 (review)

2 In suspected cases of fungal skin infection, skin or nail scrapings can be digested in 30% potassium hydroxide and microscopy of the slide preparation may confirm the infection. The same technique may be used to provide a positive diagnosis of scabies, using skin scrapings obtained after applying 10% potassium hydroxide over a suspected burrow. However, an evaluation of this technique in general practice revealed that GPs identified only 57% of the infections identified by laboratory personnel. On the basis of the figures for diagnostic accuracy quoted in the article, do you think that using this technique merits the time it would take in your surgery? Give reasons for your answer. (*2 or more points*)

Br J Gen Pract. **45**: 349–51

BMJ. **311**: 272

3 What information would you expect to find contained in the following table based on a study of treatment of tinea pedis?

BMJ. **307**: 645

	Terbinafine cream, bd for 1 week	Clotrimazole cream, bd for 4 weeks
Mycological cure rate at 4 weeks (%)	?	?
Cost (£) in 1993	?	?

Eczema pruritus and urticaria

1 Eczema. (*True/False*)

a Groups of erosions or vesicles are a regular feature of uncomplicated eczema.

b Steroid creams are less likely to provoke allergic reactions than are ointments.

c Glaucoma is a possible complication of treatment with steroid applications.

d A 3-month trial of evening primrose oil is justified in cases that resist conventional treatment.

BMJ. **310**: 843–7

2 Eczema.

a How are wet bandages best applied to an affected infant? (*2 points*)

b Avoidance of house-dust mite avoidance has been shown to make a difference to the outcome. (*True/False*)

BMJ. **316**: 1226–9 (review)

3 The following are recognized causes of pruritus ani: (*True/False*)

   a uraemia

   b psoriasis

   c uncontrolled diabetes

   d lichen planus

   e threadworms

   f ulcerative colitis

   g pediculosis

   h hyperhidrosis.

BMJ. **305**: 575–7

4 Urticaria.

   a Which antidepressant is effective against itch when applied topically as a 5% ointment?

   b Which drug class is particularly likely to cause chronic urticaria?

   c What novel treatments have been found to be successful in treating patients whose urticaria is associated with an IgG autoantibody which cross-links IgE receptors on mast cells? (*3 points*)

BMJ. **311**: 1615–17 (review)

5 The following treatments are reported to be of benefit sometimes for treatment of pruritus associated with polycythaemia:

   a cimetidine

   b aspirin

   c pizotifen

   d nifedipine

   e PUVA

   f iron.

BMJ. **310**: 580

6 Urticaria.

   a What stimuli may provoke a physical urticaria?

   b How can one determine whether a patient with relevant symptoms and a family history of severe urticaria with angio-oedema has hereditary angio-oedema?

   c What question and what test will determine whether someone has urticarial vasculitis?

d If the result of the test for urticarial vasculitis is positive, what underlying problems should be investigated, and what treatments may be offered?

e What proportion of urticaria sufferers have a dietary cause convincingly identified on double-blind challenge testing in the authors' experience?

f Of what advantage is it to a patient with chronic urticaria to have autoantibodies demonstrated against epitopes expressed on the extracellular portion of the alpha subunit of the high-affinity IgE receptor? (*2 points*)

g What medicines are particularly likely to make chronic urticaria relapse? (*3 points*)

h What form of cream is helpful for urticaria?

i What form of topical treatment is helpful for oral angio-oedema?

j If oral antihistamines are ineffective for urticaria, what oral adjunct is likely to be helpful? (*1 point*)

BMJ. **316**: 1147–50 (review)

Sunshine

1 What percentage of British holiday-makers get sunburnt when they go on package tours?

BMJ. **311**: 1062–3 (original research)

2 Protection against sunlight. (*True/False*)

a UVA radiation has no harmful effects on skin.

b Sun protection factors for sunscreens refer to protection against UVB radiation.

c There is good evidence that melanoma is related to exposure to UVB radiation rather than UVA radiation.

BMJ. **308**: 1682–6

3 Treating sunburn. (*True/False*)

a Topical steroids are indicated in mild cases.

b Oral steroids are indicated in severe cases.

BMJ. **309**: 587–9

4 An adult man with a history of excessive sweating and heat exhaustion on strenuous exercise in a hot climate has been found to have an abnormally high sweat sodium concentration and to carry mutations for cystic fibrosis genes. What implications does this have for routine practice? (*2 or more points*)

BMJ. **310**: 579–80

Skin cancer and melanoma

 1 What advice should patients be given on self-checking for skin cancer?

BMJ. **304**: 746–9, 1012–15

 2 Why may it be important to a patient that a skin lesion that has been excised is also examined histologically? (*2 points*)

BMJ. **316**: 778–9 (correspondence)

3 List three features of a mole that indicate a need for surgical biopsy.

BMJ. **301**: 1005–6

4 What clinical features of a mole would suggest that it is dysplastic? (*4 points*)

BMJ. **314**: 1438

5 Which of the following policies do you think might improve the effectiveness with which we diagnose melanoma at acceptable cost?

a Advising patients on how to identify whether they are in a high-risk group.

b Training primary care staff in the accurate visual identification of suspect skin lesions that justify biopsy.

c Inviting high-risk patients to an instruction session on prevention of melanoma and identification of suspect skin lesions.

d Sending all patients with suspect skin lesions to a dermatology clinic for a decision on whether or not to take a biopsy.

BMJ. **316**: 34–9 (survey report and discussion)

Psoriasis

1 Drugs that may aggravate psoriasis include: (*True/False*)
a beta-blockers
b sulphonamides
c NSAIDs
d chlorpromazine
e lithium
f chloroquine.
BMJ. **303**:829–35

2 What surgical operation may help recurrent guttate psoriasis?
BMJ. **312**: 1176 (citation)

3 Conventional sunbeds are a suitable treatment for psoriasis in the community. (*True/False*)
BMJ. **303**:829–35

4 A smoker with psoriasis who stops smoking will notice a distinct improvement in his psoriasis. (*True/False*)
BMJ. **308**: 428–9

5 Calcipotriol treatment for psoriasis: (*True/False*)
a takes several months to achieve maximal effect
b may cause irritation at and around the sites where it is applied.
BMJ. **305**: 847

ANSWERS

Skin treatments – miscellaneous

1 • 20% aluminium chloride applied at night, but it makes the hands sticky.
   • Oral diltiazem or anticholinergic drugs.
   • Iontophoresis of glycopyrronium bromide, but this requires attendance at the physiotherapy department.
   • Botulinus toxin.
   • Sympathectomy, but the problem may recur after a few years.

2 Thymoxamine, nifedipine and anti-inflammatory gels. Avoid exposure to cold. Chilblains on the hands are sometimes helped by exercising the arms with a windmill action to increase blood flow to the hands by centrifugal force.

3 False.

4 Chamomile cream, arachis oil, zinc and castor oil ointment.

5 a Half a gram. The area of one side of two hands.
   b About 35 grams.

6 Removing a sticking plaster may injure such skin.

7 • Dichlorvos strips (Yapona) placed in a room at night – with closed doors as it is an irritant, especially to cats – can be recommended to eliminate fleas from air and carpets.
   • A derris bath for dogs is messy but effective.
   • A flea collar is effective for cats.

8 Clingfilm.

9 Keep well away from naked flames for the next 20–30 min after applying the lotion.

10 Disease-modifying treatments:
   • steroid creams (especially useful early in the course of the condition)
   • PUVA (especially useful early in the course of the condition)
   • dermabrasion
   • mini-autologous skin grafting.

   Camouflaging treatments:
   • camouflage cream
   • tattoos
   • bleaching with hydroxyquinolines (Fade out).

Protective treatment:

- sunscreen.

11 a i Metronidazole.

ii Antihistamines, chlorpromazine, cholestyramine, cimetidine, phenobarbitone, rifampicin. Possibly ondansetron if itch is due to cholestasis.

b i Colloid or hydrogel dressing.

ii Calcium alginate dressing.

iii Potassium permanganate soaks.

Acne

1 a False.

b True.

c True.

d False – but this can occur with oral minocycline and from topical retinoids.

e True.

2 a False.

b False.

c True.

3 True.

4 Severe depression, psychosis and suicide.

5 Pigmentation – either grey due to iron deposition, or brown due to melanin deposition. It occurs in about 3.7% of users, starting on average after 5 months of treatment.

6 Chronic active hepatitis, eosinophilic pneumonitis, systemic lupus erythematosus and arthralgia.

Skin infections

1 Herpes, staphylococci, streptococci, tinea, microsporum.

2 a 7%.

b 37%.

3 Shampoo and conditioner.

4 a True.

b False – the true figure is around 60%.

c False – cases are more common in winter and spring, especially April and May.

d True.

e False – the true figure is around 10%. Fetal blood transfusion may be required.

f True.

Fungal infections

1 a Tioconazole paint twice daily or amorolfine paint weekly.

   b Tioconazole paint twice daily or amorolfine paint weekly.

   c Terbinafine 250 mg orally daily for 3 to 6 months.

   d Itraconazole 200 mg daily for 3 months.

2 The proposition that GPs examine skin scrapings and scabies burrows under the microscope met with near universal condemnation from members of Doctors' Reading Club. Several members commented that they had never convinced themselves that they had seen a scabies burrow. Since the treatments for fungal skin infections and scabies are cheap and relatively free of toxicity, prescription on the basis of clinical appearance seemed to be justified. The GP can later send a skin scraping to the laboratory if there is an unsatisfactory response to treatment.

3

	Terbinafine cream, bd for 1 week	Clotrimazole cream, bd for 4 weeks
Mycological cure rate at 4 weeks (%)	93.5	73.1
Cost (£) in 1993	4.98	4.26

Eczema pruritus and urticaria

1 a False – they indicate herpes infection.

   b False – they contain preservatives.

   c True.

   d True.

2 a A layer of moistened Tubifast and an overlying layer of dry Tubifast, or Ichthopaste or Quinaband, can be used to occlude the area.

b True.

3 a False.

b True.

c False.

d True.

e True.

f False.

g True.

h True.

4 a Doxepin.

b NSAIDs.

c Plasmapheresis, intravenous immunoglobulin and cyclosporin.

5 a True.

b True.

c True.

d False.

e True.

f True.

6 a Touch, heat, cold, sunlight.

b By assay of the fourth component of complement.

c Ask whether the weals persist for longer than 24 h, and perform a biopsy.

d Investigate for SLE or other autoimmune phenomena and for renal involvement. Treatment may be with dapsone, colchicine or oral steroids.

e 0.6–0.8%.

f Patients with these antibodies constitute 25–30% of cases of chronic (more than 6 weeks) urticaria. They can be treated effectively with plasmapheresis or immunoglobulin infusions.

g NSAIDs, opiates and ACE inhibitors.

h 1% menthol in aqueous cream.

i 2% ephedrine spray.

j A short course of steroids.

Sunshine

1 17%.

2 a False – it darkens and ages the skin and may produce ocular damage.

b True.

c False.

3 **a** True.

   b True.

4 The *BMJ* presented a case history of a soldier who developed heat-stroke after running in hot climates and who was subsequently found to have a high sweat sodium and chloride content and to carry two of the eight mutations associated with cystic fibrosis. He was azoospermic, but lung and pancreas function were normal. Members of the Doctors' Reading Club suggested that this might have the following implications for routine practice.

   Patients with cystic fibrosis may need to be reminded of the need to avoid outdoor exercise in hot weather and to drink isotonic fluid in large quantities if exposed to warm temperatures.

   Patients with heat exhaustion should have their electrolyte levels checked and if they are found to be abnormal, appropriate replacement therapy is indicated. Men with heat exhaustion and abnormally low serum sodium and chloride levels under minimal provocation may undergo sweat analysis and semen analysis and be advised thereafter.

   Genetic counselling may be indicated for those found to have the abnormal gene, but on the basis of this evidence it would appear unlikely that they would be parents to a child severely handicapped by cystic fibrosis.

Skin cancer and melanoma

1 Check for any change in size, shape or colour of birthmarks and moles. Use a mirror or ask a friend if you have a birthmark or mole on an area of skin you cannot see easily. Show the doctor any new marks which persist for longer than 2 weeks on areas of skin that are exposed to the sun.

2 To check for complete excision if the lesion is malignant, and to obtain forewarning of the need to check for other lesions if that lesion is malignant or premalignant.

3 A change in size, shape or colour. Minor features that may indicate a need for biopsy include crusting, bleeding, sensory change, and a diameter of more than 7 mm.

4 A diameter of more than 2 mm and two or more of the following: variable pigmentation, irregular asymmetrical outline or indistinct borders.

5 Most members favoured advising patients on how to identify whether they fall into a high-risk group for melanoma. Since the damage is often done very early in life, mothers might be advised of the need to keep their fair-skinned babies well covered up in sunny weather. The increased anxiety and number of patients attending with suspect lesions might be justified by the lower risk of real damage.

   Training primary-care staff in the accurate identification of lesions that justify biopsy was also favoured. Many women in particular will be happier showing their suspect freckles and naevi to a practice nurse, or may reveal them incidentally during a

Well-Woman check. Most practice nurses will already be familiar with how to identify lesions that justify biopsy, but this should be made a mandatory part of their training.

About half of the members favoured inviting high-risk patients to an instruction session on prevention and detection of melanoma. Others suggested limitations such as time pressures, low motivation among patients, and an exaggerated response by 'the worried well'. It was considered that hiring a video to relevant patients and their partners would be a good idea.

Opinion was also divided as to whether to send all patients with suspect skin lesions to a dermatology clinic for a decision on whether or not to biopsy. The biopsy can be performed with minimal fuss at the GP's surgery provided that he or she does not grudge the time it takes. Plastic surgeons usually excise melanotic lesions with a margin of about 2 mm, but if histology is positive, they commonly go back to make a wider excision. The effect of a misdiagnosis before the first biopsy is negligible provided that the biopsy is sent for histology.

Psoriasis

1 a True.
  b False.
  c True.
  d False.
  e True.
  f True.

2 Tonsillectomy if it is related to recurrent streptococcal sore throats.

3 False – difficulty in controlling the dose, as well as the danger of keratoses and skin cancers, limits their usefulness.

4 False – but a heavy drinker might well notice an improvement if he stops drinking.

5 a False (2–3 weeks).
  b True.

DIABETES

Aetiology and demographics

1 Insulin resistance is associated with: (*True/False*)

a ovarian hyperandrogenism

b beta-blockers

c congestive cardiac failure

d alpha-blockers

e ACE inhibitors

f moderate alcohol consumption.

BMJ. **313**: 1385–9 (review)

2 The following treatments increase insulin resistance: (*True/False*)

a beta-blockers

b thiazides

c calcium antagonists

d hydrallazine.

BMJ. **303**: 730–1, 755–9 (research report)

3 Vitamin E. (*True/False*)

a Low circulating levels are associated with increased risk of NIDDM even after allowing for the effects of confounding factors.

b 100 mg/day has been shown to improve glucose tolerance in healthy subjects.

BMJ. **311**: 1124–6 (original report)

Diagnosis, assessment, screening and monitoring

1 What artefact may invalidate a fingerprick blood glucose reading?

Br J Gen Pract. **44**: 42 (letter)

2 How would you interpret these laboratory results from a patient who is not taking any treatment? HbA_{1c} 10.5% and fasting blood glucose 4.2 mmol/L.

BMJ. **305**: 635–7 (case reports)

3 A 45-year-old man has a fasting blood glucose level of 6 mmol/L.

a What further test result is needed to evaluate his condition?

b If he has impaired glucose tolerance, what further follow-up is required?

BMJ. **312**: 264–5 (leading article)

4 What clinical features of a middle-aged or elderly person newly presenting with diabetes suggest a need for insulin treatment? (*2 points*)

BMJ. **310**: 1117–18 (case reports)

5 What policies are justified in order to achieve earlier diagnosis of non-insulin-dependent diabetes mellitus?

BMJ. **304**: 1154–5

6 Patients who have clinical features suggestive of diabetes may be able to self-test for glycosuria. How might you encourage them to do this at your practice? (*2 points*)

BMJ. **308**: 611, 632–5 (leading article)

7 A practice in Dewsbury sent Diastix to patients over 50 years of age who were not known diabetics, with instructions on use after a meal, and asked them to return the results to the GP. What yield of new diagnoses of diabetes would you expect from this screening procedure?

Br J Gen Pract. **47**: 371–3 (research report)

8 When screening patients aged 45–70 years not previously known to have diabetes:

a what percentage of patients would you expect to comply with a request to post back the result of a home test for glycosuria?

b of those who returned the result, what percentage would you expect to have glycosuria?

c of those with glycosuria who underwent a glucose tolerance test, what percentage would you expect to find to be diabetic?

d of those found to have diabetes, what percentage would you expect to have a fasting blood glucose level which is diagnostic of diabetes?

BMJ. **303**: 696–8 (research report)

9 Self-monitoring of diabetes.

a What are the purposes of self-testing? (*3 points*)

b What advantage does Diabur-Test 2000 have over Diastix?

c What advantage does Clinitest have over dipstick systems?

d Under what circumstances should a diabetic monitor blood glucose?

e What advice on timing of blood tests is appropriate for a non-insulin-dependent diabetic?

f What advice on timing of blood tests is appropriate for an insulin-dependent diabetic?

BMJ. **314**: 964–6 (education and debate)

10 Glycated haemoglobin level is a better predictor than blood pressure of diabetic nephropathy. (*True/False*)

BMJ. **311**: 973–7 (original article)

11 The following are useful predictors of the rate of advance of non-proliferative retinopathy in young adult diabetics: (*True/False*)

a blood pressure

b glycosylated haemoglobin

c urinary albumin excretion.

BMJ. **304**: 19–22 (research report)

Self-management

1 When monitoring diabetes: (*True/False*)

a blood glucose testing at home leads to better results on HbA_{1c} tests than does urine testing

b blood glucose test strips can be recommended for an elderly diabetic.

BMJ. **306**: 332

2 What points are worth stressing when teaching a patient how to carry out home monitoring of blood glucose? (*5 points*)

BMJ. **305**: 1171–2,1194–6 (research report)

3 What mode and style of delivering advice on controlling diabetes seems most likely to be successful with adult-onset diabetics who are not fluent in English?

Br J Gen Pract. **47**: 301–4 (project report)

BMJ. **305**: 1171–2,1194–6

4 Insulin which has been kept in a cool place becomes inactive shortly after its 'use before' date. (*True/False*)

BMJ. **313**: 58 (personal view)

5 List four or more factors that tend to make diabetes 'brittle' during adolescence.

BMJ. **303**: 260–1 (leading article)

6 A Muslim on your list controls his diabetes with an oral hypoglycaemic. He fasts in daylight hours during Ramadan. How will you advise him to adjust his oral hypoglycaemic treatment? (*1 point*)

BMJ. **307**: 292–4 (letter)

7 An insulin-dependent diabetic who controls the condition intensively so as to maintain near normoglycaemia throughout the day: (*True/False*)

a is likely to gain weight

b is at more risk than other diabetics of losing his or her driving licence as a result of the effects of hypoglycaemia

c will develop complications of diabetes substantially less quickly than other diabetics.

BMJ. **307**:881–2 (leading article)

8 The home-sharing relatives of diabetic patients are commonly more aware of the patients' hypoglycaemic attacks than are the patients themselves. (*True/False*)

BMJ. **310**: 440 (survey report)

9 Lactating mothers with insulin-dependent diabetes: (*True/False*)

a will have a higher than usual requirement for insulin

b should take the extra carbohydrate required in the morning.

BMJ. **311**: 877 (letters)

Medical management

1 What advantages do GPs have over hospital doctors with regard to the continuing care of diabetics?

Br J Gen Pract. **305**: 279–81 (survey report)

2 What biochemical assay(s) may reveal a contraindication to metformin? (*1 point*)

BMJ. **307**: 1056–7 (case reports)

3 What treatment(s) should a GP have available for treating hypoglycaemia?

BMJ. **304**: 1283–4 (survey report)

4 What precaution is needed for patients on metformin who require an X-ray with a contrast medium?

BMJ. **315**: 690 (citation)

5 In the management of hypoglycaemia: (*True/False*)

a blood glucose level is the best guide when deciding whether treatment is needed

b intramuscular glucagon takes more than 5 min to take effect

c glucagon is ineffective in hypoglycaemia induced by alcohol

d a dose of glucagon is the only treatment needed in most cases.

BMJ. **306**: 600–1 (leading article), 998 (letter)

6 Giving aspirin to prevent thrombosis in diabetics: (*True/False*)

a reduces proteinuria

b slows progression to end-stage renal disease

c slows the progression of retinopathy

d reduces the risk of heart attack in those at high risk.

BMJ. **311**: 641–2 (editorial)

7 A normoglycaemic hypertensive is found to have microalbuminuria. How will this finding affect your management of the patient?

BMJ. **304**: 1196–7 (leading article)

Complications

1 The diabetic retina. (*True/False*)

a The retinae of newly diagnosed adult diabetics are only rarely abnormal.

b Venous dilatation is a serious sign of impending loss of vision.

c Looped veins indicate a need for intense surveillance.

d Exudates at the macula are an indication for photocoagulation.

e New vessels commonly arise at the margin of the optic disk.

f Vitrectomy may salvage vision after a retinal haemorrhage.

g Aspirin is indicated for advanced retinopathy.

h Retinopathy progresses more slowly during pregnancy.

BMJ. **307**:195–8 (review)

2 Retinopathy may worsen when diabetic control improves. What are the possible reasons for this? (*2 points*)

BMJ. **315**: 1105–6

3 The following are useful predictors of the rate of advance of non-proliferative retinopathy in young adult diabetics: (*True/False*)

a blood pressure

b glycosylated haemoglobin

c urinary albumin excretion.

BMJ. **304**: 19–22

4 What proportion of patients who are registered blind as a result of diabetic retinopathy would you expect to have been having regular eye checks?

BMJ. **314**: 238 (citation)

5 What is the minimum technique for reliable assessment of diabetic retinopathy? (*2 points*).

BMJ. **311**: 207–8 (leading article)

6 You could expect the following findings from photographs of the retinae of diabetics, taking three 35-mm transparencies from overlapping areas of each retina after dilatation: (*True/False*)

a a 14% prevalence of sight-threatening abnormalities

b maculopathy is the commonest form of sight-threatening abnormality revealed

c photography has high sensitivity for maculopathy

d photography has high sensitivity for other features of retinopathy.

BMJ. **311**: 1131–5 (original research)

7 A diabetic should be advised to take the following measures to care for his feet. (*True/False*)

a Apply a plaster promptly if a sore develops under the ball of the foot.

b Use a hot-water bottle to maintain the circulation to the feet at night.

c Use bedsocks to maintain the circulation to the feet at night.

d Walk barefoot to maintain the function of the small muscles in the feet.

e Wash the feet daily.

BMJ. **303**: 1053–5 (review)

8 What rate of congenital abnormality would you expect to find in the offspring of diabetic mothers:

a who were offered routine diabetic care before and during pregnancy

b who attended a special pre-pregnancy and pregnancy diabetic clinic where diabetes was closely monitored with HBA_{1c} and preprandial blood glucose levels?

BMJ. **301**: 1070–4 (research report)

ANSWERS

Aetiology and demographics

1 a True.
  b True.
  c True.
  d False.
  e False.
  f False.

2 a True.
  b True.
  c False.
  d True.

3 a True – there was a 3.9-fold increase in risk of abnormal glucose tolerance test 4 years after the sample was taken for vitamin E assay if the result was below median.

  b False – this was demonstrated for healthy and diabetic subjects at a dose of 900 mg/day. Most vitamin E supplement pills from health-food shops contain about 200 mg per capsule.

Diagnosis, assessment, screening and monitoring

1 Sugar on the finger either because the patient has been holding a sweet or, as in this case, because they have recently vomited.

2 Haemoglobinopathy – usually persistent haemoglobin F. A high HbA_{1c} with a normal fasting blood glucose might occasionally be found in a diabetic who has recently consumed a lot of alcohol without food to accompany it.

3 a Two-hour blood glucose 2 h after taking 75 g of glucose. A result between 7.8 mmol/L and 11.1 mmol/L indicates impaired glucose tolerance.

  b An annual check on fasting blood glucose and other coronary risk factors and fundi. When diabetes is diagnosed, 16% of patients have coronary artery disease and 30% have retinopathy. However, only a minority of patients with impaired glucose tolerance go on to develop diabetes.

4 Weight loss and ketonuria.

5 The article in the *BMJ* suggested that only about 7% of diabetics are completely free of relevant symptoms at diagnosis, and the median interval between onset of relevant symptoms and diagnosis is 6–12 months. The authors also report that only 5% of the population are aware of the significance of thirst and polyuria. However, their survey provides an incomplete picture. A comprehensive study would include a survey of the symptoms and diabetic status of the catchment population. The available evidence suggests that earlier diagnosis could be achieved in many cases by a public awareness campaign in the media, including channels of communication open to GPs in leaflets and waiting-rooms. The study recorded that presentation of relevant symptoms might not result in a test for glycosuria or blood sugar. Doctors and nurses need to be more aware of the importance of testing if thirst, polyuria, weight loss, tiredness, thrush, balanitis, visual or neural disturbance or recurrent soft tissue infections are reported. Overweight people, the elderly, alcoholics and victims of self-neglect might be targeted for particular vigilance.

6 Provide patients with information on the common symptoms of diabetes in practice leaflets, posters on waiting-room walls and videos screened in waiting-rooms. Patients could be encouraged to self-test, but once they are in the GP's surgery it might be just as easy to have the urine specimen tested by the practice nurse.

7 Eight diagnoses were obtained from 1736 patients screened, at a cost of £78.25 per diagnosis.

8 a 79%.
   b 3.1%.
   c 25%.
   d 65%.

9 a   i To provide patients with information on which to base adjustments in their diet or medication.
       ii To provide the nurse or doctor with evidence on which to base advice.
       iii To detect hypoglycaemia.
   b It takes longer but the timing is less critical.
   c The large volume of colour can be seen by someone with impaired vision.
   d Blood glucose should be monitored by younger diabetics, individuals with unpredictable activities, when planning pregnancy, during pregnancy, during illness, and when first diagnosed.
   e Before breakfast, and 2 h after the main meal on 1 or 2 days per week.
   f Test before meals and at bedtime on 1 or 2 days per week, or test daily at different times. Occasional tests in the middle of the night may be useful.

10 False.

11 a False.
    b True.
    c False.

Self-management

1 **a** False.

   b False.

2 For most diabetics most of the time, tests for preprandial glycosuria combined with regular checks of HbA_{1c} suffice for monitoring their control. Blood glucose tests are needed for diabetics who are adjusting their treatment or who have a varying life-style and who wish to achieve good control without provoking hypoglycaemia. Selecting subjects capable of the procedure is the first consideration. They need to be well motivated, capable of understanding the procedure, and able to adjust their treatment in the light of the result. They also need good eyesight and the ability either to discriminate between colours on the side of the bottle, or to calibrate and use meters. It may take up to half an hour to teach them how to perform and interpret the test. A follow-up consultation will be needed within a few days to clear up any misunder-standings and to check whether home fasting levels resemble clinic fasting levels. One generally hopes that the more 'homely' surroundings of the GP surgery are less likely than the hospital diabetic clinic to provoke white-coat hyperglycaemia. Points that require particular emphasis when demonstrating the technique include correct storage of the test strips, the time interval between applying the blood and reading the result, and regular calibration of the meter. Automatic meters are now nearly universal. They minimize the timing difficulty as they have an electronic countdown, and they also have a digital display which avoids the need to interpret colours.

3 The adviser should speak the language in which the patient is most fluent. Instruction should be given individually or in family groups, not in groups of strangers. Non-attenders should be followed up by telephone. Discuss the benefits in terms of well-being for the patient and their family, and longevity. Aim to persuade the entire household.

   A structured questionnaire may highlight areas in which the patient requires advice. The use of flashcards showing familiar household items, particularly foods and kitchen items, helps to demonstrate points, but some people may find this demeaning. At follow-up discuss the patient's experiences with the dietary changes, and estimate their compliance.

4 False – it will remain biologically active for several years if it is kept cool.

5 The following factors were listed in the reference:
   • manipulation of therapy in order to achieve the patient's desired weight
   • emotional or psychosocial problems causing irregular control
   • loss of awareness of hypoglycaemia
   • enhanced counter-regulatory responses to hypoglycaemia
   • insulin resistance due to high growth-hormone levels during adolescence.

Further factors suggested by doctors who have answered this question included:
- poor doctor–patient communication
- obsessive attention focused on maintaining a blood glucose level in the normal range
- poor insulin absorption because the same injection site is used every time
- denial of the problem because of social pressures.

6 Take the main dose of the oral hypoglycaemic at sundown.

7 a True.
  b True.
  c True.

8 True.

9 a False – their insulin requirement is likely to remain unchanged.
  b False – the mother should drink an extra pint of milk and consume an extra 50 g of carbohydrate, preferably late in the day when she is most likely to be hungry.

Medical management

1 They are more accessible, with better timekeeping and more interest in the patient's home circumstances.

2 Serum creatinine or urea. Renal failure contraindicates metformin.

3 Lucozade or some other glucose drink, glucagon, and possibly intravenous glucose.

4 They should stop metformin for 48 h before and 48 h after taking the contrast medium.

5 a False – it correlates poorly with symptoms.
  b True – the author misquoted the reference.
  c True.
  d False – glucose is then needed to replenish the hepatic stores.

6 a True – but this may be due to altered renal haemodynamics rather than to a protective effect.
  b False.
  c False – the overall impression gained from clinical trials is that there is no slowing in the progression of retinopathy and no reduction in the risk of retinal haemorrhage.
  d True – aspirin is indicated for those with a history of heart attack, angina or thrombotic stroke or transient ischaemic attack if there are no contraindications. It would also be valid to consider treatment for those with microalbuminuria, old age or standard risk factors for ischaemic heart disease.

7 Consider the use of ACE inhibitors for blood pressure higher than 140/80 mmHg.

Complications

1 a False.

   b False.

   c True.

   d True.

   e True.

   f True.

   g False.

   h True.

2 It is possibly due to a drop in blood flow or a rise in secretion of growth factor (IGF_1) from the liver when normoglycaemia is restored. Uncontrolled diabetics with retinopathy should undergo any necessary laser treatment before a major improvement in diabetic control is introduced.

3 a False.

   b True.

   c False.

4 About half according to this report.

5 According to this article, ophthalmoscopy and retinal photography through dilated pupils, performed by experienced personnel.

6 a True.

   b True – about three times more common than other forms of sight-threatening abnormality.

   c False – a figure of 61% is quoted, but the addition of photographs centred around the macula might improve this.

   d False – a figure of 47% is quoted. However, false negatives on this feature commonly had maculopathy which was observed from the photographs. The overall number of false negatives from this form of screening is acceptably low, and much better than the number obtained with direct ophthalmoscopy performed by untrained personnel.

7 a False – support around the sore rather than directly over it is what is needed.

   b False – there would be a risk of scalds to numb feet.

   c False – the risk of athlete's foot is increased.

   d False – there would be a risk of sores to numb feet.

   e True.

8 a 10%.

   b 1.5%.

ENDOCRINE, METABOLIC AND BONE DISEASE AND LIPID DISORDERS

Endocrine disorders

1 When assessing thyroid function: (*True/False*)
a intercurrent illness affects TSH values but not T_4 values
b glucocorticoids reduce total T_4 values and TSH values, but do not affect thyroid status
c T_3 levels are useful in the investigation of possible hyperthyroidism but not in that of possible hypothyroidism.

BMJ. **307**: 177–9

2 Screening for hypothyroidism.
a Which subgroup of pregnant women is particularly susceptible to autoimmune thyroiditis postpartum?
b Which drug treatments may cause hypothyroidism?
c Which non-thyroid cancer is associated with Hashimoto's thyroiditis?
d How much commoner is subclinical hypothyroidism in individuals with increased total cholesterol than in those with normal cholesterol levels?

BMJ. **314**: 1175–8 (review)

3 List three endocrine causes of male impotence. (*3 points*)

BMJ. **307**: 275–6

4 The following have been reported as presenting features of Addison's disease: (*True/False*)
a vitiligo
b jaundice
c xanthopsia
d confusion

e vomiting.

BMJ. **312**: 1085–6 (case reports)

5 What are the clinical features of growth hormone deficiency of adult onset? (*4 points*)

BMJ. **313**: 314 (leading article)

6 Testosterone deficiency.

a What symptoms or signs may justify screening a 60-year-old man for testosterone deficiency? (*3 or more points*)

b If testosterone deficiency is found, what contraindications are there to replacement therapy? (*5 points*)

BMJ. **313**: 1214 (book review)

Metabolic disease

1 With what endocrine disorders may haemochromatosis present? (*5 points*)

BMJ. **316**: 915–16 (case reports)

2 A conscientious man suffers no hangover on Sunday morning after a drinking session on Saturday night, but he does note fatigue on Monday morning after heavy drinking on a Saturday. Relatives have experienced a similar problem. What might it be, and what treatment helps?

BMJ. **316**: 871 (anecdote)

Obesity

1 Factors in obesity. (*True/False*)

a Increasing food intake explains the recent increase in obesity in the UK.

b A high intake of sugar is associated with obesity.

c Social classes 4 and 5 have a higher energy intake than social classes 1 and 2.

d Social classes 4 and 5 have a higher fat intake than social classes 1 and 2.

BMJ. **311**: 437–9 (discussion paper)

2 The following naturally occurring agents or medicines are likely to lead to increased food intake: (*True/False*)

a dopamine

b glucagon

c noradrenaline

d opioids

e serotonin.

BMJ. **315**: 997–1000 (review)

3 The following conditions in an obese woman are likely to improve while she loses weight: (*True/False*)

a infertility

b gallstones

c hyperuricaemia

d polycystic ovary syndrome.

BMJ. **303**: 704–6

4 Prevention of obesity may be accomplished more effectively by public policy and law than by exhorting individuals. What policies seem genuinely likely to make a difference and also to be politically acceptable? (*3 or more points*)

BMJ. **315**: 477–80 (education and debate)

5 Waist circumference may be a suitable measurement with which to assess the degree to which overweight is contributing to patients' risk of thrombotic disease. Are there any adjustments to the observation or validation studies you would wish to see before adopting it into your practice? (*3 or more points*)

BMJ. **311**: 158–61

6 Men with a waist circumference of 94 cm (37 inches) are very likely to have a body mass index of 30. (*True/False*)

BMJ. **311**: 1401–5 (original research)

7 What forms of treatment have been shown to be practicable and effective in the treatment of obesity? (*3 points*)

BMJ. **307**: 577–8
BMJ. **309**: 654–6

8 Match the following items of advice to overweight patients to the descriptions:

  i relatively effective for weight reduction

  ii relatively ineffective for weight reduction

  iii may be useful for selected patients.

  a take more exercise

  b involve the whole family in buying, cooking and eating food with more fibre and fewer calories

  c try to eat less and drink less alcohol

  d join a slimming club

  e use a precise diet and calorie-counting method

  f observe and modify your eating behaviours

  g read a leaflet that gives details of good eating habits

  h keep a diary of body weight and food consumption.

  Br J Gen Pract. **41**: 147–9

9 Obese people are best advised to diet constantly until they reach the target weight for their height. (*True/False*)

  BMJ. **313**: 1225 (news item)

Metabolic bone disease

1 By how much does thiazide treatment reduce the rate of bone loss in elderly men?

  BMJ. **301**: 1303–5

2 The following observations are associated with effects on forearm bone density in premenopausal women: (*True/False*)

  a history of a fracture

  b history of breast-feeding

  c body mass index

  d serum alkaline phosphatase

  e use of a thiazide diuretic

  f serum calcium.

  Br J Gen Pract. **41**: 194–6

3 For each of the following statements about prevention of osteoporotic fractures indicate whether you think it is true or false, and give a reason for your point of view.

   a Bone density is a valuable predictor of risk to the individual.

   b Taking hormone replacement treatment from the age of 50 to 65 years will substantially reduce the cumulative lifetime risk of a fracture for a woman.

   c Daily physical exercise for 1 h confers about 50% protection.

   d Stopping smoking reduces the risk by about 25%.

   e An annual supplement of calciferol is indicated for elderly women.

   f Decreasing salt intake will reduce the risk.

   BMJ. **303**: 453–9, 920–2

4 Osteoporosis induced by long-term use of depot medroxyprogesterone acetate is irreversible. (*True/False*)

   BMJ. **308**: 247–8

5 At what time of life will a high calcium intake have most effect on bone mass in late adulthood? (*1 point*)

   BMJ. **309**: 930–1

6 In later life an increase in bone mass is an accurate index of a decrease in bone fragility. (*True/False*)

   BMJ. **309**: 931–2

7 Hip fractures in Indian people. (*True/False*)

   a Hip fractures are more common in elderly Indian women than in elderly white women.

   b Hip fractures are more commonly subtrochanteric (and therefore likely to be related to osteomalacia) in Indian people than in white people.

   BMJ. **309**: 1124–5

8 Biphosphonates: (*True/False*)

   a have been shown to reduce fracture rates in postmenopausal osteoporosis

   b are the treatment of choice for Paget's disease

   c once started, treatment should be continued *ad infinitum*.

   BMJ. **309**: 711–15

9 **a** What condition renders patients particularly susceptible to the side-effects of long-term treatment with alendronate or pamidronate?

b What instruction should be given to patients using these drugs?

BMJ. **315**: 1235 (letter)

10 As well as measures to increase bone mass, what else can be done to reduce the risk of fractures related to osteoporosis in elderly people? (*3 or more points*)

BMJ. **310**: 950, 989–92

11 A patient with a clinical condition that places him or her in a high-risk category for osteoporotic fracture should undergo bone densitometry before starting treatment. Do you agree with this statement? State reasons and limiting factors for your point of view. (*2 or more points*)

BMJ. **310**: 1507–10

Nutrition

1 What intake of the following is suggested by Government dietary recommendations?

a Portions of fruit or vegetables per day.

b Portions of potato, pasta or rice per day.

c Portions of fish per week.

BMJ. **309**: 1323 (summary report)

2 Supplements of which nutrients may be indicated for someone with prolonged vomiting?

BMJ. **305**: 517–18, 891

3 Low tissue concentrations of which nutrient are associated with an increased incidence of pressure sores?

BMJ. **305**: 925–7

4 On the basis of present evidence, which children in the UK may justifiably be prescribed supplements of vitamin A? (*4 points*)

BMJ. **306**: 366–70

5 What nutrients are most likely to be required as dietary supplements by vegans? (*5 points*)

BMJ. **306**: 804

BMJ. **314**: 1834 (letter)

6 Roughly how many of the UK population receive fluoride in their water supply?

BMJ. **306**: 1481

7 Some cases of restless leg syndrome can be cured by correcting a deficiency of which nutrient? (*1 point*)

BMJ. **307**: 880

8 Which nutrient may halve the incidence of senile macular degeneration? (*1 point*)

BMJ. **309**: 1452 (citation)

9 What are the nutritional disadvantages of fruit squash as the only fluid consumed by a young child? (*3 or more points*)

BMJ. **310**: 486

10 How many milligrams of elemental iron would you expect to find in 100 g of vegetable curry after it has been cooked in a cast-iron balti wok?

BMJ. **310**: 1368

11 Selenium. (*True/False*)

  a Dietary intake in Europe has been falling.

  b A daily supplement of about 1 mg/day is appropriate.

  c Low serum concentrations are associated with a significantly higher risk of spontaneous abortions.

  d Sperm motility has been observed to improve with supplementation.

  e Cancer mortality fell by 5% in individuals receiving selenium supplements compared to those receiving placebo.

BMJ. **314**: 387–8 (leading article)

12 What appears to be the optimal dose of supplemental vitamin E for enhancing immune function in the elderly?

BMJ. **314**: 1369

13 Against what condition does a high intake of coffee appear to provide protection?

BMJ. **315**: 1388 (citation)

14 List several good dietary sources of folic acid. (*5 points*)

BMJ. **316**: 498 (news item)

Lipid disorders

1 What effect does an intercurrent minor infection have on serum cholesterol? (*2 points*)

BMJ. **315**: 1244 (citation)

2 Moderate alcohol consumption in women is likely to have the following metabolic effects: (*True/False*)

a reduces total triglycerides

b reduces total cholesterol

c reduces insulin sensitivity.

BMJ. **304**: 80–2

3 By how much does a cup of filter coffee per day raise serum cholesterol levels?

BMJ. **311**:1582 (citation)

4 In Finnish men the presence of serum IgG antibodies to *Chlamydia pneumoniae* has been found to be associated with higher levels of serum triglyceride and lower levels of HDL cholesterol. What may account for this? (*2 or more points*)

BMJ. **314**: 1456–7 (research report)

5 Hypercholesterolaemia is much more common in people with other risk factors for coronary heart disease. (*True/False*)

BMJ. **302**: 1057–60

6 In a cohort of middle-aged men in the UK you could expect the following risk factors to change significantly over 12–13 years: (*True/False*)

a body weight

b blood pressure

c total cholesterol

d total triglyceride.

BMJ. **303**: 678–81

7 The British Hyperlipidaemia Association currently recommends that measurement of serum cholesterol in healthy people be restricted to those who have xanthomas or arcus senilis, or a history or family history of atherosclerosis at an early age. (*True/False*)

BMJ. **302**: 605–6

8 What appears to be the best index of hypercholesterolaemia for prognostic purposes?

BMJ. **315**: 1554–5 (leading article)

9 A patient is found to have hyperlipidaemia on screening. What steps would you take to exclude the possibility that it is secondary to an underlying cause? (*3 points*)

BMJ. **309**: 509–10

10 Which patients with hypercholesterolaemia should be tested for hypothyroidism? (*2 points*)

BMJ. **308**: 918

11 What are the recommendations of the British Hyperlipidaemia Association on use of lipid-lowering therapy in patients with pre-existing coronary artery disease? (*3 points*)

Br J Gen Pract. **48**: 983–4 (survey report)

12 There is good evidence that the following patients will benefit from treatment to lower their serum cholesterol: (*True/False*)

a a survivor of a myocardial infarct with a serum cholesterol level of 6 mmol/L

b a patient with no history or symptoms of coronary heart disease, but with a serum cholesterol level of 7 mmol/L.

BMJ. **310**: 1280–1

13 Dietary treatment to lower plasma cholesterol levels achieves its maximal effect by 3 months. (*True/False*)

BMJ. **301**: 1377

14 A practice has a policy of advising patients with a serum cholesterol level of more than 5.5 mmol/L to follow a low-cholesterol and low-fat diet, to keep their weight to below a body mass index of 25 kg/m^2 and to substitute unsaturated for saturated fats. Following this policy, approximately what percentage reduction in serum cholesterol can be expected in the following groups of patients in the long term?

    a Compliant patient with serum cholesterol level of less than 6.5 mmol/L.

    b Average patient with serum cholesterol level less than 7.5 mmol/L.

    c Compliant patient with serum cholesterol level more than 7.5 mmol/L.

    d Average patient with serum cholesterol level more than 7.5 mmol/L.

BMJ. **303**: 953–7

15 What is a likely cause of resistance to HMG CoA reductase inhibitors, and how may this factor be measured? (*2 points*)

BMJ. **316**: 1127–30 (research report)

16 What effect would you expect guar gum, 5 g three times per day, to have on low density serum cholesterol levels?

BMJ. **310**: 95–6 (research report)

17 What dose of dried garlic will reduce serum triglyceride and cholesterol levels by an average of 10–15%?

BMJ. **303**: 379, 785

18 When serum cholesterol levels drop, any reduction in cardiac mortality is offset by an increase in non-cardiac deaths. Can you suggest one or more hypotheses to explain this finding?

BMJ. **303**: 3–4

ANSWERS

Endocrine disorders

1   **a** False.
     b True.
     c True.

2   **a** Insulin-dependent diabetics, who should be tested for thyroid antibodies in the first trimester.
     b Lithium and amiodarone. Users of these drugs should be tested for thyroid function annually.
     c Breast cancer.
     d Two- to threefold.

3   Diabetes, testicular failure and hyperprolactinaemia.

4   **a** True.
     b False.
     c False.
     d True.
     e True.
     The list of possible presenting features of Addison's disease includes weakness, anorexia, malaise, hyperpigmentation (particularly of the gingival mucosa, scars and skin creases, and present in 92% of cases), vitiligo, postural hypotension, abdominal pain, nausea, vomiting, diarrhoea, constipation, myalgia, arthralgia, confusion, psychosis and depression. Adrenal crisis is characterized by rapid onset of hypotension, tachycardia, fever and hypoglycaemia and a progressive deterioration in mental status.

5   Fatigue, depression, midline obesity, thin skin and osteoporotic fractures.

6   **a** Fatigue, loss of libido and loss of muscle mass.
     b Prostate cancer, heart failure, hypertension, polycythaemia and sleep apnoea.

Metabolic disease

1   Women may develop amenorrhoea. Men may develop hypogonadism. Either sex may develop diabetes.

2   Familial periodic paralysis. Potassium supplements.

Obesity

1 a False.

   b False.

   c False.

   d False.

2 a False.

   b False.

   c True.

   d True.

   e False.

3 a True.

   b False – supersaturation of bile is more likely as body stores of cholesterol are mobilized.

   c True.

   d True.

4 Government might attempt to counter obesity by the following measures:

   - taxing fattening foods and alcohol
   - teaching the benefits of healthy eating to schoolchildren
   - having health visitors teach healthy homecraft to parents
   - reducing the fat content of school meals
   - prominent labelling of the calorie content of foods
   - subsidising supervised slimming clubs
   - encouraging people to take more exercise.

   Exercise might be promoted by providing more cycle routes, cycle-loan schemes in town centres, leisure centres, allotments, supervisors to accompany children as they walk to school, pedestrianizing more streets and housing areas, and taxing use of the private car and using this money to subsidise public transport.

5 Waist circumference correlates closely with body mass index and is more sensitive to changes in intra-abdominal fat, which is associated with heart disease. Adjusting for height did not improve the strength of the correlation. A waist circumference of more than 102 cm for men or 88 cm for women identified 98% of people with a BMI of more than 30. The public would find it easier to measure their waist circumference or read it off their clothing than to calculate their body mass index without a table. Asking patients about their waist circumference could be an easy way of assessing whether they need to slim and advising them on acceptable limits. However, doctors would find it more difficult and less acceptable to measure waist circumference than

to measure height and weight. Obese people will find it no easier to reduce their waist circumference than their weight.

6   False. For men a waist circumference of 94 cm (37 inches) corresponds to a BMI of more than 25 or a high waist-to-hip ratio. A waist circumference of 102 cm (40 inches) corresponds to a BMI of more than 30 or a high waist-to-hip ratio. For women a waist circumference of 80 cm (32 inches) corresponds to a BMI of more than 25 or a high waist-to-hip ratio. A waist circumference of 88 cm (34 inches) corresponds to a BMI of more than 30 or a high waist-to-hip ratio.

7   Professor Garrow in his article in the *BMJ* pointed out that the only treatment for obesity that has been shown to be effective is self-financed but non-profit-making slimming groups, run by dietitians, using a combination of calorie-counting and increased energy output to achieve a loss of 0.5 to 1 kg per week. However, his comments are challenged by those who point out that 90–95% of individuals who lose weight put it back on again afterwards. The lifelong need to control food intake must therefore be emphasized to patients.

Several members made further suggestions. Dietitians often concentrate on the calorie and nutrient content of foods. Perhaps therapists for obesity might enjoy more success if they also dealt with the emotional and behavioural aspects of eating, in particular using cognitive therapy and hypnotherapy to improve self-esteem, discussion of alternative ways to prevent or to relieve tension, alternative sources of comfort and pleasure, and suggesting distraction techniques to use when tempted to comfort-eat.

One doctor suggested that self-discipline is an unrealistic expectation for many people. Those who lack it may benefit from developing an image of a source of benign discipline within their minds.

Involving other members of the household in helping the obese person to lose weight also seems worthwhile. Their behaviours while shopping, preparing food, eating and tidying away the remaining food will greatly influence the temptation to overeat.

8   The following answers are based on a consensus of GPs responding to this question:
    a may be useful for selected patients
    b relatively effective
    c relatively ineffective
    d relatively effective
    e may be useful for selected patients
    f relatively effective
    g relatively ineffective
    h relatively ineffective.

9   False. A structured programme of 3 months of weight loss, followed by a period of stabilization while the brain readjusts to the lower weight, followed by a further period of weight loss is more likely to be adhered to. Other points alluded to in this report from the Scottish Intercollegiate Guidelines Network Working Party include more widespread use of appetite-controlling drugs, and involvement of the whole family.

Metabolic bone disease

1   Thiazide treatment is reported to reduce bone loss in elderly men by 29–49%.

2   **a** True.
     b False.
     c False.
     d True.
     e True.
     f False.

3   The authors of this paper argued that bone density, while a valuable measure of the efficacy of preventive treatment, is of little value in determining risk to the individual, as hip fractures are mainly incurred in falls and accidents which are random independent events. The distributions of bone density in individuals with and without hip fracture show extensive overlap. However, bone density appears to be useful for selecting those who will benefit from prophylaxis. Measures to reduce the incidence of falls in the elderly are also likely to be important.

     The authors cited references reporting that metacarpal bone density declines to the values found in untreated controls in the 4 years after hormone replacement treatment (HRT) is stopped, and that hip fracture rates increase to those found in untreated controls in the 5 years after HRT is stopped. Correspondents cited a reference which reported that differences in forearm bone density between controls and treated populations are maintained after stopping HRT. The balance of evidence suggests that stopping HRT at the age of 65 years would have little effect on fracture rates in women in their late seventies and eighties, the age group in which most fractures occur.

     The authors cited trial evidence that walking protects against hip fractures only, but a programme of regular physical exercise three times a week confers about 50% protection against fractures at all sites. However, there are problems of compliance with this advice.

     Stopping smoking before the menopause would confer 25% protection against fracture.

     Evidence does not yet support the introduction of vitamin D supplements to prevent osteoporotic fractures. However, reducing sodium intake to 70 mmol/day (4 g of salt) reduces calcium excretion by about half the deficit observed in menopausal women with an average intake of calcium. Thiazide diuretics have a similar effect, and prolonged use of these drugs has been associated with a significant reduction in hip fractures.

     A high content of calcium in the diet has a modest effect in reducing osteoporosis. Skimmed milk, cottage cheese, yoghurt and sardines seem to be the best sources.

4   False – such bone loss does reverse when medroxyprogesterone treatment is stopped.

5   Before the age of 25 years, and preferably before puberty.

6   False – once trabeculae have been destroyed, adding mineral to those that remain will not add commensurate strength to the bone.

7   a False.

     b True.

8   a False.

     b True.

     c False.

9   a A history of dyspepsia.

     b These patients should not lie down shortly after taking the dose.

10   Help them to develop and maintain their strength, co-ordination and general health, treat visual impairment, treat alcoholism, treat postural hypotension, and minimize use of sedatives. Use hip protectors. Provide walking aids and grab rails. Eliminate loose mats and obstructions on walkways.

11   Doctors responding to this question were divided as to whether to prescribe treatments that prevent osteoporosis in the absence of bone densitometry findings. Techniques for measuring bone density are still being developed and assessed, and there are only about 160 scanners in the NHS. Inevitably there are delays and long distances for patients to travel if all of them are to be screened. The risk of fracture increases by a factor estimated to be between 1.5 and 3.3 for every standard deviation in the distribution of results, but possibly a discriminant function based on observations from the history and examination would be almost as powerful a predictor. Insufficient studies have been reported that relate the efficacy of treatments in reducing fracture rates to the results of densitometry at different ages. Until this information is available we will have to use guesswork.

Nutrition

1   a 6.

     b 3.

     c 2.

2   Thiamine and phosphate.

3   Vitamin C.

4   Infants with very low birthweight, babies with malabsorption and acute or chronic infection, and babies with cystic fibrosis or AIDS who are prone to infection. Doses of supplements should be close to the recommended daily allowance.

5   Iron, riboflavin, iodine, vitamin B_{12} and selenium.

6   Six million. Knowing the fluoride content of water in your locality will affect the advice you offer to parents on whether their children should take fluoride supplements.

7 Iron.

8 Carotenoids found in green leafy vegetables.

9 Excess intake of refined sugar, and therefore dental caries, dependence on sweet foods, reduced intake of more varied nutrients, and excess swings in blood sugar level. Tartrazine sensitivity is another disadvantage.

10 10.6 mg – a useful tip for vegetarians.

11 a True.

b False – supplements of more than 800 mcg/day are toxic. A daily dose of 200 mcg is about right.

c True – this was shown in a recent UK study.

d True – in a double-blind controlled trial an improvement from 17.5% to 35.1% was noted.

e True – this occurred in a randomized trial.

12 200 mg/day.

13 Cancer of the colon.

14 Folate is found in fortified cereals, orange juice, bananas, whole grains, and leafy green vegetables such as spinach.

Lipid disorders

1 It depresses it by about 4%.

2 a True.

b True.

c False.

3 Each daily cup raises cholesterol by only 0.05 mmol/L. Cafetiere coffee, in which the grounds are mixed with the boiling water for longer, probably raises the cholesterol level further.

4 Chlamydia multiply inside macrophages, leading to the production of cytokines, particularly interleukin 1 and tumour necrosis factor. These may increase serum lipid levels.

5 False.

6 a True.

b False.

c True.

d False.

7   False – they recommend that all men should have their cholesterol checked in early adult life.

8   The ratio of total cholesterol to HDL cholesterol.

9   When the GP authors of the original study screened some 300 patients with cholesterol levels higher than 6.5 mmol/L, the exercise yielded one unexpected case of hypothyroidism, two of diabetes, three to five cases of raised gamma-GT suggestive of excess alcohol intake, and four possible cases of renal failure. Most doctors responding to this question thought it worth bearing these underlying causes of hyperlipidaemia in mind when a raised lipid level is reported. It seems unnecessary to screen these patients for hypothyroidism or alcoholism on this evidence unless they have suggestive clinical features on examination and history-taking. However, diabetes and renal failure are additional risk factors for arteriosclerosis and may lead to treatment being modified. A check on whether they have been ruled out does therefore appear to be justified.

10 Hypothyroidism is associated with low-density hypercholesterolaemia and no significant hypertriglyceridaemia. The level of LDL cholesterol at which it is worth testing for hypothyroidism may depend on the patient's clinical presentation, but a high index of suspicion is needed if the level is significantly raised (a total cholesterol level of more than 7.8 mmol/L).

11 Introduce a lipid-lowering agent if the serum cholesterol level is more than 5.2 mmol/L and there is pre-existing coronary heart disease or two other risk factors, and only after a strict dietary regime lasting 3 months.

12 a True – the cut-off point for using lipid-lowering drugs in this group currently seems to be around 6 mmol/L if 3–6 months of dietary counselling have failed.

    b False – accepted cut-off point for lipid-lowering drugs in this group is 7.8 mmol/L.

13 False.

14 a 8%.

    b 1%.

    c 12%.

    d 3%.

15 If the raised cholesterol value is due mainly to cholesterol derived from gastro-intestinal absorption rather than synthesis in the body, HMG CoA reductase inhibitors are likely to be relatively ineffective. The ratio of cholestanol to cholesterol is an index of the proportion of cholesterol derived from the diet.

16 Guar gum at this dose is reported to reduce low-density lipoprotein cholesterol levels by about 10% after 1 year of use and by about 20% after 2 years of use.

17 800 mg/day.

18 Follow-up studies suggest that lowering lipids does not bring about the expected benefits to survival. Instead there has been an excess of accidental deaths in those with lower lipids levels. This may be a statistical anomaly, but there are a number of

alternative explanations. Are those who comply with dietary advice and take their tablets a self-selected group? Are they more ill than the non-compliant patients? These seem unlikely explanations, as the overall lack of benefit is found in randomized studies analysed by intention to treat. Is randomization to an active intervention group a stress factor in itself, causing malnutrition, hypoglycaemia or fitness fanaticism? Does sequestering cholesterol in the gut cause bowel disease? Does the reek of garlic provoke violence from companions? Results from subsequent studies suggest that this finding of increased mortality in patients who lower their cholesterol levels may be spurious and due to a statistical anomaly.

EPILEPSY

Diagnosis and assessment

1 The following clinical features of an episode of loss of consciousness suggest an epileptic seizure rather than a syncopal attack: (*True/False*)
  a the attack happening within seconds of a blow to the head
  b brief jerking or stiffening of the extremities as the person loses consciousness
  c the vision going grey before the attack
  d a guttural cry as the attack commences
  e cyanosis
  f irregular breathing
  g pelvic movements and back arching
  h recovery of consciousness within a minute.
  BMJ. **314**: 158–9 (leading article)

2 What features are useful for differentiating a pseudoseizure (a conversion symptom) from a genuine fit? List four or more.
  BMJ. **301**: 1331

3 Chance of recurrence.
  a If a patient has a single epileptic seizure, what is his chance of suffering a recurrence, assessed on the day of the seizure?
  b If the patient with a single seizure is first seen and assessed 1 month later, what is the likelihood of his suffering a recurrence?
  BMJ. **301**: 1112–14

4 In a patient with a single seizure, the following factors are associated with an increased likelihood of recurrence: (*True/False*)
  a the single seizure was nocturnal

b the single seizure happened just before a menstrual period

c the patient is aged over 40 years

d there is a family history of epilepsy or febrile fits.

BMJ. **302**: 620–3, 102-3

5 A young adult who has had a single seizure during an alcoholic hangover is very unlikely to have an underlying neurological lesion demonstrated on investigation. (*True/False*)

BMJ. **309**: 986–9

6 In epilepsy: (*True/False*)

a seizures characterized by sudden loss of muscle tone have a good prognosis

b provoked seizures have a good prognosis

c patients with generalized grand mal epilepsy should have a magnetic resonance brain scan.

BMJ. **301**: 1112–14

BMJ. **302**: 363–6

7 A 16-year-old youth has been seen to jerk violently on wakening on two occasions a few months apart. What investigation(s) will you arrange?

BMJ. **305**: 4–5
BMJ. **304**: 1416–19

8 A toddler went pale, fainted and his whole body shook for about 30 s after an immunization. He recovered consciousness after a few minutes. A similar sequence of events happened when he fell down some steps. What is the prognosis? (*2 points*)

BMJ. **307**: 214–15

9 What is the diagnosis and prognosis for children who suffer attacks described as follows?

a A preschool child suffers pallor, coma, stiffening and opisthotonos for about 30 s after tripping and falling while running.

b A 2-year-old has a generalized tonic-clonic fit lasting about 5 min while feverish with a flu-like illness.

c A child aged between 2 and 12 years with no family history of epilepsy and who is developing normally starts to suffer seizures affecting the tongue, face and arm when he wakes up in the morning.

d An intelligent 10-year-old child with no family history of epilepsy has lapses of attention and memory for a minute or two every 2 weeks.

e A 6-month-old baby has had several attacks when he flexes his trunk in spasm every 5 to 10 s and stops paying attention to his surroundings.

f A 5-year-old who is a slow developer has a history of several types of seizure, including absence attacks, muscle jerks, and going limp, with long periods of paralysis and inattention thereafter.

g A hitherto normal 2-year-old fails to develop socially and now barely speaks, and starts to suffer seizures of several types.

BMJ. **315**: 924–30 (review)

Management

1 What would you regard as suitable criteria for the following aspects of good medical care of patients with epilepsy? (*6 or more points*)

a Documentation of seizures and use of medication.

b Frequency of planned review.

c Indications for laboratory studies.

d Indications for review of medication.

Br J Gen Pract. **46**: 731–3 (audit report)

2 Can you suggest a check-list of points on which all epileptic patients should receive advice?

Br J Gen Pract. **46**: 11–14 (research article)

3 What appear to be the main areas of difficulty in the care of people with epilepsy in the community. (*5 points*)

Br J Gen Pract. **46**: 37–42 (review)

4 A 16-year-old youth has been seen to jerk violently on wakening on two occasions a few months apart. What advice will you give the youth?

BMJ. **304**: 1416–19

BMJ. **305**: 4–5

5 What advice do you give your epileptic patients on how to avoid seizures? (*5 points*)

Br J Gen Pract. **93**: 453–6

6 A patient has had epileptic seizures both by day and by night. When can he obtain a driving licence? (*2 points*)

BMJ. **310**: 885–6

7 Why is extra vigilance needed when monitoring epilepsy in a young adult?

BMJ. **316**: 339–42 (follow-up study)

8 What criteria should prompt referral of an epileptic for consideration of neurosurgical treatment? (*3 points*)

BMJ. **313**: 383 (news item)

Treatment

1 In epilepsy: (*True/False*)
  a if a patient feels tired, dizzy and sick after 1 week on treatment with phenytoin at the recommended introductory dose, another drug should be substituted
  b sodium valproate is the drug of first choice for a patient with primary generalized seizures
  c the dose of sodium valproate should be monitored by serum levels
  d carbamazepine may be better tolerated if given in a slow-release formulation.

BMJ. **302**: 363–6

2 If a combination of two drugs is needed to treat epilepsy, it would seem sensible to combine drugs of different classes. To which classes do the following drugs belong?
  a carbamazepine
  b lamotrigine
  c phenytoin
  d sodium valproate
  e vigabatrin.

BMJ. **315**:885 (letter)

3 When monitoring phenytoin treatment of epilepsy: (*True/False*)
  a ataxia is the most sensitive clinical sign of toxicity
  b plasma levels are directly related to dose

c the sample should be taken 12 h or more after the last dose

d the drug is only effective at plasma levels of 40–80 mmol/L

e concomitant use of sodium valproate makes plasma levels difficult to interpret

f folic acid increases blood levels of phenytoin.

BMJ. **305**: 1215–18

ANSWERS

Diagnosis and assessment

1 a False – this suggests a concussive convulsion with a benign prognosis.
  b False.
  c False.
  d True.
  e True.
  f True.
  g False – this suggests a pseudoseizure.
  h False.

2 Gaze aversion, resistance to passive limb movement or eye opening, prevention of the hand falling on to the face, induction by suggestion, and normal serum prolactin levels during an attack.

3 a 60–80%.
  b 40–60%.

4 a True.
  b False.
  c False.
  d True.

5 True.

6 a False.
  b True.
  c False – However, a magnetic resonance brain scan is justified for those with focal or temporal lobe epilepsy.

7 Neurologists regard the diagnosis of epilepsy as clinical rather than based on EEG with provocation or on brain scan. A clear history of jerking on two occasions would justify treatment if consciousness was also impaired. If the jerking was bilateral without loss of consciousness, the diagnosis would be myoclonic jerks. Unilateral jerking at an age when cerebral tumour is a relatively likely cause of the problem justifies the search for an epileptic focus.

8 These attacks are reflex anoxic seizures. They may recur with sudden traumatic events until the child is aged 5–12 years, but they do not indicate epilepsy.

9 a These are white reflex asystolic attacks. In the absence of any adverse features such

as history of trauma or family history of epilepsy, or any developmental delay they are likely to be self-limiting and the prognosis is excellent.

b In the presence of the adverse factors listed above, about 10% of children with fever fits, especially those whose fits are prolonged, go on to develop epilepsy. In most children the prognosis is excellent.

c These seizures from a Rolandic focus are usually benign, but they require control with anti-epileptic treatment, and some sufferers have associated neuropsychiatric features.

d In the absence of adverse features or other types of seizure, the outlook for sufferers of these petit mal seizures is good.

e Infantile spasms have a poor prognosis, but treatment with corticosteroids or vigabatrin may be effective.

f This is Lennox Gestaut syndrome and the prognosis is poor.

g This is Landau Kleffner syndrome and the prognosis is poor.

Features suggestive of a poor prognosis for children's seizures include family history, early onset, additional neurological impairment, onset without a history of provocations such as fever, head injury, meningitis or hypernatraemic dehydration, multiple types of seizure, frequent or long seizures, and poor response to anti-epileptic drugs.

Management

1 Eliminating seizures or at least minimizing their frequency allows epileptics to lead more independent lives. However, some of them despair of controlling the problem and suffer needlessly, or are rendered inactive by two side-effects of treatment. GPs may need to take the initiative in ensuring that these patients are followed up and receive the best possible treatment and advice.

Most doctors answering this question considered that epileptics should record each seizure as it occurs and present their diaries or tell the GP about the event at an appointment within the next week. Epileptics who are free of seizures on treatment may benefit from a reminder every year or two that the GP expects to be told of any seizure that occurs. This will require a register of patients on anti-epileptics. Only if we set high standards can we influence the quality of control.

Prescribing and use of medication should be recorded at each consultation, and since some epileptics have poor memories for drug names, they may need reminding to bring the tablets or their treatment card with them. It is realistic to expect that most epileptics can be controlled by the use of one or two drugs taken once or twice daily. Patients on phenytoin, carbamazepine, primidone and phenobarbitone require drug level measurements if they suffer somnolence or are seen to have ataxia, slurred speech or nystagmus on lateral gaze or have an isolated fit or an increased frequency of fits, or if a further treatment is introduced that may have a pharmacokinetic interaction with the anti-epileptic.

Patients on carbamazepine require full blood counts and liver function tests before initiation and after a few months of using the drug. Those on phenytoin or phenobarbitone require annual full blood counts and either serum calcium and alkaline phosphatase or else serum vitamin D measurement to check for impending osteomalacia.

Review of medication is indicated if fits are increasing in frequency, if the patient is finding the treatment intolerable, if the treatment is interacting unpredictably with another necessary treatment, if the patient wishes to start a family, or if the treatment is inappropriate (e.g. carbamazepine for generalized seizures).

2 The author of the original article suggests the following points: compliance with medicines, side-effects of medicines, use of alcohol, and self-help groups.

The patient should be warned to avoid prolonged fasting, undersleep, drinking to excess, driving, swimming and bathing until further advice has been given.

Psychological issues include the following:

- probable benign prognosis
- coming to terms with the diagnosis
- side-effects of treatment
- lack of effect on employment prospects
- lack of effect on longevity.

3 The findings of the reviewer reporting in the *British Journal of General Practice* were as follows:

- lack of systematic follow-up
- inappropriate polypharmacy
- patient non-compliance with medication
- failure of GP–patient communication
- low levels of patient knowledge.

4 Doctors answering this question suggested starting the patient on valproate and advising him that lifelong treatment may be needed. The news might be softened by pointing out that we are all prone to seizures if sufficiently provoked, and that controlled epilepsy is common and carries no stigma. The only occupational restrictions are the police, the armed forces and occupational driving.

There is a need to avoid hazards such as drowning and falling from a height until seizures are controlled, and also the risk of fits when hungry, dehydrated or overtired, or during a hangover. An identification bracelet can be carried by poorly controlled epileptics, but would appear to be unnecessary in this case. The information on self-care might need to be discussed during a series of consultations.

5 The common precipitants of seizures are missed doses of anti-epileptic treatment, fatigue, hangover, hunger, fever, stress, hypoxia at altitude, and flashing lights such as may be encountered when playing computer games or visiting discotheques. Epileptics should promptly take paracetamol if they develop a feverish illness. Female epileptics are particularly vulnerable when they are premenstrual. Epileptics should be told to report fits promptly in case these suggest a need to alter the

treatment. After a fit the patient should rest and eat and remember to take the next dose of their anti-epileptic before resuming normal activities, and they should be aware that seizures sometimes occur in clusters and that they are particularly vulnerable to further fits in the next few days. Doctors answering this question also mentioned the desirability of avoiding activities which would involve particular danger if a seizure occurred, especially bathing, climbing and handling machinery at times when the patient is vulnerable.

6 After 3 years during which epileptic seizures have only occurred during his sleep, or after 1 year during which he has been free of any seizures.

7 This study found that six of 124 people with epilepsy aged up to 23 years died between the ages of 17 and 23 years, but none died before the age of 17 years.

8 In one report from America, those epileptics selected for surgery had had complex partial or secondary generalized seizures occurring monthly or more often for more than 1 year, despite trying three or more anticonvulsants. Resources are limited, so younger people should have priority.

Treatment

1 a False – tolerance of symptomatic adverse effects improves with continued use. Temporary dose reduction is appropriate.
  b True.
  c False – serum levels correlate with efficacy only for phenobarbitone, phenytoin, carbamazepine and ethosuxiside.
  d True.

2 a Sodium-channel blocker.
  b Sodum-channel blocker.
  c Sodium-channel blocker.
  d Sodium-channel blocker with GABA-ergic properties.
  e GABA transaminase inhibitor.

3 a False – nystagmus is the most sensitive sign.
  b False.
  c False – timing is not critical.
  d False.
  e True.
  f False – it reduces them.

GYNAECOLOGY

1 What treatment would you suggest for the following women with pre-menstrual syndrome?

a The patient's main symptom is breast tenderness. She is otherwise well, but has found paracetamol at the recommended dose to be ineffective.

b The patient's main symptoms are tiredness and irritability lasting for a whole week before each period for the past 6 months. She is quite content in her relationships and life-style.

c The patient gets irritable and miserable and notes breast pain and bloating before her periods. She is using Microgynon 30 as a contraceptive.

BMJ. **304**: 194

BMJ. **307**:1471–5

2 What is your differential diagnosis for the following patients with menstrual irregularities? What gynaecological investigations will you perform or request in each case? *(12 points)*

a A 25-year-old woman is becoming increasingly obese. Her periods were regular until 4 months ago, when they stopped. She hopes to have a baby and has been using no contraception for the past 4 months. A recent pregnancy test is negative. She is tense and unhappy because of marital and employment problems.

b A 32-year-old woman reports that her periods have been unusually heavy and painful for the past 4 months. She has no vaginal discharge and no dyspareunia. She is unmarried and does not require contraception. Her cervical smear 6 months ago showed no dyskaryosis or inflammatory changes.

c A 40-year-old woman has had irregular bleeding per vaginam on average for 3 days in 12 for the past 4 months. She has no vaginal discharge and no dyspareunia. She has borne three children and was sterilized by tubal ligation 5 years ago. Her cervical smear 1 year ago showed no dyskaryosis or inflammatory changes.

BMJ. **306**: 225–6

3 Some women with secondary amenorrhoea may best be treated with the combined contraceptive pill. What would be your selection criteria for identifying them? (*5 points*)

BMJ. **306**: 516

4 What percentage reduction in menstrual blood flow would you expect to find in women with menorrhagia treated with the following regimes for the first 5 days of menstruation?

a ethamsylate 500 mg qds

b mefenamic acid 500 mg tds

c tranexamic acid 1 g qds.

BMJ. **313**: 579–82 (trial report)

5 Menorrhagia.

a What hormonal treatments appear worthy of consideration for menorrhagia?

b What advantages does the levonorgestrel-containing intra-uterine device have over oral treatment in the management of menorrhagia? (*3 points*)

BMJ. **313**: 75 (letter)

BMJ. **314**: 160–1 (leading article)

6 Levonorgestrel coils are an extremely effective treatment for menorrhagia in women in their forties. What gynaecological problems caused continuation of prolonged bleeding after insertion of a coil in a minority of the subjects in this study? (*4 points*)

BMJ. **316**: 1122–5.

7 Endometrial sampling.

a Who, of the 15% of women in their forties who suffer menorrhagia, should undergo screening for endometrial cancer?

b What is the risk that a Pipelle sample will yield a negative result in a patient who has endometrial cancer? (*3 or more points*)

Br J Gen Pract. **47**: 387–90 (discussion paper)

8 A 50-year-old woman is soon to have a hysterectomy for cervical cancer. What misunderstandings may she have that could reduce her ability to enjoy future sexual relations with her partner? What advice may help the couple to re-establish their sexual relationship? (*6 or more points*)

BMJ. **308**: 869–70

9 What is the median return-to-work time in days:

    a after abdominal hysterectomy

    b after laser endometrial resection?

BMJ. **303**: 1362–4

10 What prevalence of straining at stool has been reported as a new problem after hysterectomy?

BMJ. **316**: 160 (citation)

11 What are regarded as indications for aspiration of an ovarian cyst? (*5 points*)

BMJ. **313**:1098 (editorial)

12 Endometriosis. (*True/False*)

    a It is commoner in women taking the pill.

    b It is commoner in women using the IUCD.

    c Treatment will reverse infertility.

BMJ. **306**: 158–9, 182–4

13 Subfertility.

    a For how long should a man refrain from sexual activity before providing a specimen for semen analysis?

    b In a subfertile woman with a low level of progesterone 5 days before her periods, what therapeutic inferences would you draw from the following associated features:

        i high levels of FSH and LH

        ii high levels of LH but normal FSH together with high androgen levels

        iii borderline high prolactin?

    c What treatment can be offered to a woman with endometriosis leading to tubal blockage?

    d What preparations should be made to maximize the success rate of intra-uterine insemination?

    e For what cause of infertility is *in-vitro* fertilization preferable to intra-uterine insemination?

    f What is the success rate of *in-vitro* fertilization?

    g What is the success rate of intracytoplasmic sperm injection?

Br J Gen Pract. **47**: 111–16 (review)

14 What investigations would you arrange for an infertile couple before they are seen at an infertility clinic? (*5 points*)

BMJ. **306**: 1728–31

15 In a woman who is now symptom free 2 days after what appears to be a complete miscarriage at 12 weeks, how might one assess whether she is likely to benefit from curettage? (*2 points*)

BMJ. **310**: 1426

16 Prolapse.

  a What examination techniques help to identify the condition at an early stage? (*3 points*)

  b How often should vaginal pessaries be changed?

  c What adjunct to the use of vaginal pessaries will reduce discomfort and the risk of erosion?

  d What advantages have been shown from the use of oestrogens before repair operations?

BMJ. **314**: 875–9 (review)

17 Surgery for stress incontinence.

  a If urodynamic studies indicate additional urgency or urge incontinence, surgical treatment is contraindicated. (*True/False*)

  b What proportion of those who undergo treatment report a benefit?

  c What proportion of those who undergo treatment report a cure?

BMJ. **315**: 1493–8 (survey report)

18 A considerable proportion of choriocarcinomas present after a normal birth. (*True/False*)

BMJ. **316**: 532–4 (case report)

ANSWERS

1 We need to be aware of the range of treatments available for premenstrual symptoms, as none of them enjoy predictable success. Our question therefore related to three different symptom patterns.

    a Most doctors who answered this question suggested bromocriptine for the woman with breast pain unrelieved by paracetamol. Evening primrose oil still finds some favour despite its limited efficacy in trials. Danazol was considered as a last resort because of its side-effects.

    b Tiredness and irritability in the premenstrual week are increasingly treated with a serotonin reuptake inhibitor. Progestogen supplements in the latter half of the cycle and oestrogen and progestogen sequential preparations are also worth considering. Many members would also discuss life-style, particularly relaxation techniques and sleeping, eating, smoking, drinking and exercise habits.

    c The patient who experienced irritability, misery, breast pain and bloating before her withdrawal bleeds on Microgynon 30 might benefit from using a lower-dose contraceptive on a tricyclic regime. Vitamin B_6 might be helpful for the mental symptoms, and bendrofluazide might be useful for the bloating. Alternatively, the patient could switch to a different contraceptive technique.

2 a Differential diagnosis – polycystic ovaries, stress amenorrhoea, hypothalamic-pituitary disorder.
    Investigations – FSH/LH ratio, oestradiol, progesterone, prolactin, testosterone.

    b Differential diagnosis – endometriosis, submucous fibroid, adenomyosis.
    Investigations – examine and smear the cervix, pelvic ultrasound, refer for endometrial biopsy and hysteroscopy if these services are available.

    c Differential diagnosis – dysfunctional uterine bleeding, fibroid, adenomyosis, adenocarcinoma, cervical polyp, chronic cervicitis.
    Investigations – examine and smear the cervix, pelvic ultrasound, refer for endometrial biopsy and hysteroscopy if these services are available.

3 Once pregnancy has been excluded, the commonest cause of secondary amenorrhoea is hypoestrogenaemia due to anxiety or weight loss. Restoring the cycle with a combined oral contraceptive may improve confidence and prevent bone loss. The cycle commonly returns spontaneously when treatment is stopped. However, before oestrogen treatment is started members suggested checking the woman's weight, taking a history of any recent stresses, and ruling out other causes of amenorrhoea by requesting assay of LH and FSH, androgens, prolactin and thyroid hormones and examining for virilization and ovarian cysts or tumours.

4 a 0%.

    b 20%.

    c 54%.

5 a Progestogen supplements have proved inferior to tranexamic acid in several trials. However, these authors in the *BMJ* suggest that the combined pill reduces blood loss by half, and that the levonorgestrel coil reduces it by 80–90%.

b It is more effective, more convenient, provides contraceptive care, and reduces the risk of sexually transmitted diseases.

6 Adenomyosis, fibroids, endometritis and endometrial cancer.

7 a We should concentrate screening for endometrial cancer on those who are in their fifties or very late forties, who are nulliparous, hypertensive, overweight or diabetic, and who are single or have never used a combined oral contraceptive, as these are high-risk groups. Possibly also concentrate on those who have irregular bleeding, or heavy or prolonged periods after introducing HRT, and those whose menorrhagia does not respond to standard medical treatment.

b There is a published report of 8 missed cases out of 103, as well as several cases reported as atypia rather than endometrial cancer.

8 A woman facing a hysterectomy for cervical cancer is likely to be sexually inhibited by worries about the prognosis and the rigours of the operation, possibly compounded by a needless concern that the disease is infectious, and guilt that her previous sexual encounters may have started the disease. She may also be under the misapprehension that her vagina will be removed, that her hormone balance will be affected, or that radiotherapy may be harmful to her husband. After the operation she may need to be reassured that the scar will heal fully within a few weeks and that sexual intercourse thereafter will be neither painful nor dangerous. If the couple are concerned that they are no longer able to enjoy marital relations, several options may be suggested to ease the resumption of sexual activity. Pelvic floor exercises may help to redevelop the musculature. An oestrogen cream may be useful both for its hormonal effect on the vagina and because its use encourages the woman to handle the vulva and vagina. Initially sex may need to be non-penetrative. A vibrator or vaginal dilator and lubricant may help the couple. However, a sensitive GP broaching the topic will try to avoid giving a middle-aged couple the impression that they are abnormal if they do not enjoy frequent sexual intercourse.

9 a 64 days.

b 14 days.

10 In total 90 of 315 women who had hitherto been free of constipation noted an increased need to strain at stool after hysterectomy. Fifty of them had to resort to digital evacuation. In a comparison group of women who had had a laparoscopic cholecystectomy, only 5 of 58 patients reported increased difficulty in evacuating their bowels thereafter.

11 In the view of the writer of this *BMJ* editorial, in premenopausal women, a decision on whether to aspirate a relatively small ovarian cyst of benign appearance on ultrasound may be deferred for 3–6 months, as about half of them will resorb and only a small proportion, estimated at 0.3–2.3%, are malignant.

In postmenopausal women, cysts of benign appearance on ultrasound (unilocular, anechogenic, and less than 50 mm in diameter) should be aspirated as the risk of malignancy is higher. Those that have a more sinister appearance or which are associated with a CA125 above 35 IU/mL should be treated surgically.

12 a False.

    b False.

    c False.

13 a 5 days.

    b i Probable ovarian failure.

      ii Probable polycystic ovaries.

      iii Consider a dopamine agonist as the first line of treatment.

    c Operate to remove the blockage and then provide 6 months of treatment with danazol or a GnRH analogue.

    d Stimulate the ovaries with clomiphene or a similar drug. Remove sperm from the plasma of the ejaculate in order to reduce the bacterial content and to concentrate motile sperm. Time the injection to coincide with ovulation.

    e Bilateral tubal blockage.

    f Average rate is 20%.

    g Average rate is 30%.

14 Two semen analyses 3 weeks apart, luteal-phase progesterone, prolactin, full blood count and (if indicated) rubella antibodies.

Some members also mentioned the woman's weight, basal body temperature chart, thyroid function, spinnbarkeit of cervical mucus, history of pelvic inflammatory disease or gynaecological procedures, age at menarche and previous menstrual history.

15 Ultrasound may be used to show whether there are retained products of conception, and beta-HCG level is also needed to exclude the possibility of a continuing pregnancy or trophoblastic disease.

A history of continuing vaginal discharge or a finding of an enlarged uterus or tenderness on bimanual examination would also suggest a need for evacuation.

16 a Use of Sims speculum applied to the posterior wall to detect cystocoele and applied to the anterior wall to detect rectocoele or enterocoele. Palpating the vaginal walls while the patient stands and coughs may also reveal prolapse.

    b Every 6 months.

    c Oestrogen cream.

    d Oestrogen increases vaginal wall thickness and reduces the incidence of post-operative cystitis.

17 a False.

    b 87%.

    c 28%.

18 True – up to 50%.

HEREDITARY DISEASE

1 People who have a parent with Huntington's chorea, and who have taken a biochemical test to determine whether they too will suffer this in future, experience great psychic distress if the result comes back indicating a high probability. (*True/False*)

BMJ. **313**: 828 (citation)

2 Haemoglobin electrophoresis has revealed that a child is a heterozygous carrier of sickle- cell disease. What are the advantages and dangers of telling the parents this information? (*8 or more points*)

BMJ. **313**: 407–10 (review)

3 Homocystinuria.
   a What clinical features might lead you to suspect this diagnosis? (*6 points*)
   b Why is it inappropriate to take the confirmatory blood sample at the GP surgery? (*1 point*)

BMJ. **313**: 1025–6 (leading article)

4 For what possible treatment should patients with Marfan's syndrome be referred? (*1 point*)

BMJ. **307**: 507–8

5 Cascade screening for Fragile X syndrome.
   a What are the benefits of screening?
   b What information should be given when the topic is introduced?
   c Who should approach the individual family members who are to be screened?

BMJ. **315**: 1174–5, 1223–6 (leading article, project report and discussion)

6 Couples who have borne one child with cystic fibrosis generally comply with subsequent offers of prenatal diagnosis and termination of affected pregnancies. (*True/False*)

BMJ. **316**: 240 (citation)

ANSWERS

1 False – it appears that knowledge of the reality of the prognosis is no worse than worrying about the uncertainty.

2 Advantages:
- parents are then encouraged to be tested before planning future pregnancies
- the child may be advised on the risk for his or her own children, and may seek to have a partner tested before marriage
- siblings may be tested
- all carriers in the family may be informed of the risk of hypoxia, dehydration and prolonged blood-vessel occlusion by tourniquet.

Disadvantages:
- the child may be misinformed of the risk to his or her own health and develop unnecessary anxiety as a result
- the child may be stigmatized by health examiners or employers
- there may be exposure of non-paternity.

3 a Normal at birth but progressive impairment of intellect, myopia and dislocation of lenses in childhood, thromboembolic events usually starting around the age of 30 years, marfanoid features, and spinal osteoporosis in adolescence.

   b Measuring homocyst(e)ine in plasma requires a sample which is deproteinized within a few minutes of collection. However, a urine sample may be provided at the GP surgery. These tests are not completely reliable, as there are technical problems with the assay.

4 An aortic graft may prevent dissection of the aorta.

5 a The benefits of screening are as follows. Forewarning may lead to antenatal diagnosis in subsequent pregnancies if the parents are willing to consider termination of a severely affected child. The incidence of the problem is now much lower in New South Wales as a result of such a screening policy.
   Earlier diagnosis of mildly affected relatives may make it easier for them to obtain remedial teaching and psychological support. Sometimes other genetic problems can be detected earlier.

   b Presenting the problem will require sharing of understanding of the nature of the condition, the fact that it varies in severity and affects twice as many boys as girls, the nature of chromosomes, X-linked inheritance, and the fact that the condition is almost always transmitted to the next generation via the mother. The family should be asked if they know of any relatives affected in a similar manner to their own child. The child's mother and the brothers, sisters, cousins and aunts of the affected child on the mother's side of the family should all be checked if they might bear children in the future. The father should also be checked, as he may have a mild form of the condition and, if so, all of his relatives should be checked as well.

c Because of the possibility that parents will be hostile or defensive, or may be unwilling to give details of other family members, presentation of the need for screening may best be undertaken by a clinical geneticist, who can trace family members through the registry office if necessary, contact them and arrange to meet them in person, or have the local clinical geneticist do so if they live in another area.

6 False – the results of the study showed that 24 of 42 families who had a child affected with cystic fibrosis declined the offer of prenatal diagnosis at the next pregnancy, and in 8 cases they accepted a prenatal diagnosis but decided against termination.

Some members thought that this might be a result of poor communication by doctors. Others thought that it could be due to parents not recognizing the implications of the diagnosis while their child was still small, being unwilling to contemplate another pregnancy at the time when they were asked, feeling that to reject an affected fetus might appear like an act of disloyalty to their existing child, or developing fatalistic attitudes.

INCONTINENCE

1 What proportion of people over 30 years of age who suffer from incontinence would you expect to have consulted their GP about it?

BMJ. **306**: 832–4

2 What question(s) might you ask in order to assess the severity of urinary incontinence?

BMJ. **312**: 961–4 (review), 1459–62 (research report)

3 Clear descriptions of stress incontinence and urge incontinence are enough to confirm these diagnoses. (*True/False*)

BMJ. **313**: 112

4 Screening and treating for urinary incontinence.

a What prevalence of urinary incontinence (two or more leaks in any one month) would you expect in British middle-aged and elderly women?

b What cure rate would you expect in middle-aged and elderly women with urinary incontinence who were willing to undertake a supervised programme of pelvic floor exercises and bladder training?

BMJ. **303**: 1308–12

5 Incontinence in women. (*True/False*)

a Obesity is related to stress incontinence.

b Surgery for prolapse is likely to cure stress incontinence.

c Oestrogen creams may help stress incontinence.

d Training techniques for incontinence need only be used for a few weeks or months to have a lasting effect.

e Operative surgery is of benefit to most women with detrusor instability.

f A procedure involving prolonged bladder distension is of benefit to most women with detrusor instability.

Br J Gen Pract. **43**: 426–8

6 Why may stress incontinence become a coronary risk factor? (*1 point*)

BMJ. **312**: 1620 (citation)

7 An elderly woman complains of incontinence without any other relevant complaints or findings on examination. Would you treat the symptoms or refer her immediately for investigation? State reasons for your point of view.

a If the pattern of symptoms clearly suggests stress incontinence.

b If the pattern of symptoms clearly suggests urge incontinence.

BMJ. **313**: 754 (letter)

8 **a** What form of bladder training is suggested for people with detrusor instability and consequent urge incontinence?

b Would you expect this training to be markedly effective in reducing the frequency of micturition or the number of incontinence episodes?

BMJ. **302**: 994–6

9 Management of incontinence.

a What general measures could be provided or advised by a GP to control any type of incontinence?

b What measures could be taken or advised by a GP clinic to control the following types of incontinence:

  i   stress incontinence

  ii detrusor instability

  iii reflex bladder.

BMJ. **303**: 1453–6

10 How would you instruct a woman with stress incontinence on the technique of pelvic floor exercises and check that she is doing these exercises properly?

Br J Gen Pract. **41**: 445–9

11 What are the essential prerequisites for a trial of intermittent self-catheterization in an incontinent patient?

Br J Gen Pract. **305**: 253–5

12 A patient with incontinence due to a neurological handicap would like to learn the technique of intermittent self-catheterization. Where can he obtain a booklet of instruction?

BMJ. **307**: 1084

13 Faecal incontinence.

    a What are its common precursors? (*8 points*)

    b Which sufferers might appropriately be referred for which form of surgery? (*10 points*)

    c Which patients might be helped by sacral nerve stimulation? (*1 point*)

BMJ. **316**: 528–31 (review)

ANSWERS

1 83%.

2 The author suggests the following questions. How many pads (changes of underwear) do you need per day? What type of pads do you use? How often do you need to change the sheets? Ask the patient to record the frequency of micturition and the number of episodes of incontinence over 48 h.

3 False – urodynamic studies often reverse the impression gained from the history.

4 a 17% from the results of this study.

  b 11% from the results of this study.

5 a False.

  b False.

  c True.

  d False.

  e False.

  f True.

6 It deters sufferers from vigorous activity.

7 a Stress incontinence in an elderly woman can be helped by surgery, but before making a referral for this, many GPs addressing this question thought that they might encourage the use of pelvic floor exercises and oestrogen cream, and possibly Femina cones (supplied by Colgate Medical, Windsor), and check for urinary infection, and for prolapse which might justify the use of a ring pessary.

  b Urge incontinence may also be helped by bladder distension under anaesthesia, but before making a referral, several GPs addressing this question favoured a trial of bladder training, and possibly oxybutinin or one of its congeners.

    The argument against delayed referral is that urodynamic tests are easy to perform, result in the reclassification of a substantial minority of cases of incontinence, and the end results of treatment supervised by a specialist are likely to be better than those achieved by GPs working in isolation.

    Much therefore depends on the attitude of the patient and the clarity of the history and symptom pattern.

8 a Advise the patient to try to delay bladder emptying as long as possible when the urge to pass urine is noted.

  b No. Improvement over 6 weeks in this trial was only slight, with only 7 of 19 patients observing a significant improvement. Additional treatment with terodiline gave results that were only marginally better.

9 a • Advice on pads and garments.

    • Fluid restriction.

- Avoidance of excessive use of diuretics.
- Control of constipation.
- Control of urinary infection.
- Advice on smoking if there is a chronic cough.
- Oestrogen replacement.
- Pelvic floor exercises.
- Use of self-catheterization.

b i

- Pelvic floor exercises.
- Intravaginal cones.
- Maximum electrical stimulation.
- Urethral plug.
- Oestrogen and phenylpropanolamine.

ii

- Bladder training – relaxation techniques.
- Prescription of oxybutinin, imipramine, propantheline, nifedipine, phenylpropanolamine, propranolol, oestrogen or desmopressin.

iii

- Check for diabetes, hypothyroidism and use of drugs.
- Check for outflow obstruction or refer for cystoscopy.
- Instruct in self-catheterization.

10 The author suggests advising the patient to do 5–10 sessions of 10 contractions per day and to check the quality of the contraction of the sphincter muscles with two fingers in the vagina.

11 A well-motivated patient, and a bladder that retains an adequate volume of urine (over 100 mL is suggested).

12 Family Doctor Publications, 1 Northumberland Avenue, London WC2N 5BW. Price £3.50 including postage.

13 a Perineal damage at childbirth, sphincter damage at haemorrhoidectomy or sphincterotomy for fissure, multiple sclerosis, spinal injuries, spina bifida, dementia, diabetic neuropathy, radiotherapy for pelvic cancer, progressive systemic sclerosis, idiopathic intestinal pseudo-obstruction.

   b Sphincter tears can be repaired or a substitute sphincter constructed from the surrounding muscles. Anal leakage may be treated with an artificial sphincter with a fluid reservoir. Patients who are not helped by a regime of alternating enemas and constipating agents may be helped by antegrade colonic irrigation after the appendix is brought to the surface. A colostomy may be needed as a last resort.

   c Sacral nerve stimulation may help to treat neuropathic problems.

LIVER DISEASE

1 Hepatitis A.

   a What is the risk that a traveller to an underdeveloped country will contract hepatitis A?

   b What reduction of the risk is provided by using inactivated hepatitis A vaccine, and for how long?

BMJ. **311**: 1351–5 (review)

2 What would explain the following laboratory results on testing for hepatitis B?

   a Core antibody negative, surface antibody positive, surface antigen negative.

   b Core antibody positive, surface antibody positive, surface antigen negative.

   c Core antibody negative, surface antibody positive, surface antigen positive.

BMJ. **307**: 276–7

3 If a pregnant woman is a carrier of hepatitis B, what should be done? (*2 points*)

BMJ. **314**: 1033–7 (debate)

4 The persistent carrier state is more likely to develop in adults than in children who contract hepatitis B. (*True/False*)

BMJ. **311**: 1178–9 (editorial)

5 What is the estimated prevalence world-wide of chronic infection with hepatitis B?

BMJ. **308**: 146

6 Natives of which countries have a particularly high carriage rate of hepatitis B? (*5 points*)

BMJ. **312**: 507 (letter)

7 What percentage of Vietnamese immigrants were found by the author of this article to be carriers of hepatitis B?

Br J Gen Pract. **41**: 301

8 Infection with hepatitis C virus: (*True/False*)

a rarely has any long-term effect

b responds completely to antiviral chemotherapy in most cases

c can be transmitted by sexual contact.

BMJ. **306**: 469–70

9 European carriers of HBsAg are likely to develop cirrhosis within 10 years. (*True/False*)

BMJ. **306**: 530

10 One partner in a faithful relationship has hepatitis C. What advice should be given to each partner on sexual contact thereafter? (*3 or more points*)

BMJ. **312**: 357–63 (review)

11 Asymptomatic infection with hepatitis C virus.

a What is the prevalence of infection with hepatitis C virus in the community?

b What proportion of those individuals with the virus acquired in the community can be expected to develop chronic hepatitis?

BMJ. **308**: 670–1

12 Hepatitis C. (*True/False*)

a Interferon treatment is best provided early in the course of the disease.

b Most patients who are seropositive are aware that they have hepatitis.

c Injecting drug-users should be tested for the condition.

BMJ. **311**: 1187–8 (news)

13 Your practice nurse pricks herself accidentally with a needle that has been in the arm of a patient. What would you do? (*4 points*)

BMJ. **309**: 989–90

14 Hepatitis E: (*True/False*)

a is much more common in tropical than temperate climates

b has a dangerous chronic phase

c may cause mortality in late pregnancy

d almost always confers lifelong immunity

e is mainly spread by blood and saliva.

BMJ. **310**: 414–15

15 In a patient with jaundice, what laboratory specimen is required to detect hepatitis E virus?

BMJ. **302**: 399

16 Ursodeoxycholic acid is of proven benefit for alcoholic cirrhosis of the liver. (*True/False*)

BMJ. **301**: 1291

17 Liver tumours causing obstructive jaundice are always resistant to therapy. (*True/False*)

BMJ. **314**: 333 (case report)

18 What other autoimmune condition is associated with primary biliary cirrhosis? (*1 point*)

BMJ. **316**: 562 (citation)

19 Primary biliary cirrhosis. (*True/False*)

a It can be treated.

b It is associated with rheumatoid arthritis.

c The first symptom is usually painless jaundice.

d It has a support group.

e Anti-microsome antibodies are a specific test for the condition.

BMJ. **312**: 1181–2 (leading article)

20 What treatments are available for bleeding oesophageal varices in patients with cirrhosis that is not advanced?

BMJ. **316**: 1320 (letter)

ANSWERS

1 a 3–20/1000 per month.

  b Over 95% for 10 years.

2 a This patient has received hepatitis B vaccine.

  b This patient has been infected with hepatitis B and is immune.

  c This patient is a hepatitis B carrier.

3 The infant should have hepatitis B immunoglobulin at birth and three doses of hepatitis B vaccine.

4 False – babies born to mothers who are e antigen positive and who contract the infection have a 60–90% chance of becoming chronic carriers. Such infection can be prevented by immunizing babies actively at birth if their mothers are seropositive. About 0.74% of mothers can be expected to harbour the infection, judging from data from The Netherlands. About 27% of mothers are screened for hepatitis B at antenatal clinics.

5 5%.

6 China, Hong Kong, Malaya, Vietnam and Singapore.

7 17%.

8 a False – over half of the patients develop chronic hepatitis.

  b False – less than half of the patients respond to inteferon alpha, and many of these relapse when treatment is withdrawn.

  c True.

9 False.

10 There is no need for barrier methods. However, sexual contact during or just after menstruation should be avoided. The partner should be tested regularly for hepatitis C antibodies. Condoms should be used for any casual sexual contact.

11 a 1/1400.

  b About 14%.

12 a True.

  b True (but one-third of the patients in this study were unaware).

  c True.

13 The first priority is to minimize the risk of transmission of infection, so washing, antiseptic, and magnesium sulphate paste to draw serum from the wound are useful. GPs addressing this question suggested taking blood from the patient in whose arm the needle had previously been, to check (with his permission) for hepatitis B and C antigens and HIV antibodies. The nurse could also be tested for hepatitis B antibodies immediately and again around 4 months later.

Human normal immunoglobulin should be given immediately and hepatitis B immunoglobulin ordered for administration to the nurse if the patient is HBsAg positive. If the nurse is HBsAb negative, hepatitis B active immunization is also indicated. Procedures to prevent recurrence of needlestick injuries also need to be checked.

14 a True.
    b False.
    c True.
    d False.
    e False.

15 Stool for electron microscopy. No serological test is yet available.

16 True.

17 False – occasionally, as in this case, the tumour is a lymphoma which is extremely responsive to chemotherapy.

18 Coeliac disease – 3% of patients with coeliac disease had biliary cirrhosis, and 6% of patients with biliary cirrhosis had coeliac disease.

19 a True – ursodeoxycholic acid improves symptoms and delays complications.
    b True.
    c False – it is usually lethargy.
    d True – the PBC Support Group can be contacted at The Liver Trust, Central House, Central Avenue, Ransomes Europark, Ipswich IP3 9QG.
    e False – antimitochondrial antibodies are a specific test.

20 Subcutaneous octreotide, 100 mcg tds for 15 days, oral beta-blockers and sclerotherapy.

NEUROLOGY

Diagnosis

1 What observations on physical examination are most likely to lead to diagnosis of a cerebral tumour in a young person with a persistent headache? (*2 points*)

BMJ. **315**: 996 (anecdote)

2 The Babinski response is a reproducible clinical sign in the vast majority of patients in whom it is found. (*True/False*)

BMJ. **304**: 482

3 What clinical features would help to differentiate a complex partial seizure from a panic attack? (*5 points*)

BMJ. **306**: 709.

4 How is syringomyelia likely to present?

BMJ. **316**: 189 (personal recollection)

5 Benign paroxysmal positional vertigo.

  a What position of the head is used to test for this condition?

  b How long does the condition typically persist?

  c What form of training may improve the condition? (*3 points*)

BMJ. **307**: 1507–8

6 What are the symptoms and signs of normal pressure hydrocephalus in an adult? (*3 points*)

BMJ. **309**: 750

7 In a 60-year-old man, leg tremor while erect, relieved for a short time by walking a step, is most probably due to alcoholism. (*True/False*)

BMJ. **310**: 143–4 (editorial)

8 A patient appears to have Bell's palsy. What should you do to rule out Ramsay Hunt syndrome before giving steroids? (*2 points*)

BMJ. **315**:1163

9 Why should lumbar puncture needles have a round end?

BMJ. **315**: 1324 (leading article)

10 Multiple sclerosis is extremely unlikely in the following groups. (*True/False*)

a Immigrants from India and Pakistan who arrived when over the age of 15 years.

b Immigrants from India and Pakistan who arrived during childhood.

c Caribbean immigrants.

BMJ. **315**: 1388 (citation)

11 How does the variant form of Creutzfeldt-Jakob disease present? (*5 points*)

BMJ. **316**: 563–4 (leading article)

12 What form of sensory loss has been found in keyboard users in a preliminary study? (*1 point*)

BMJ. **316**: 575 (news item)

13 Channelopathies.

a When a channelopathy causes a gain in function, what are the typical clinical features? (*3 points*)

b When a channelopathy causes a loss of function, what the are typical clinical features? (*3 points*)

BMJ. **316**: 1104–5 (editorial)

14 Reflex sympathetic dystrophy. (*True/False*)

a It is due to excess catecholamines at the site of injury.

b Osteopenia is found in most chronic cases.

BMJ. **310**: 1645–9

Management

1 What circumstances would lead you to ask for immediate admission because you suspect a patient has malignant cord compression?

BMJ. **316**: 18–21 (prospective study report)

2 What surgical procedure can pre-empt aspiration of food and drink in a patient with long-term paralysis of the swallowing mechanism?

BMJ. **304**: 459–60

3 When botulinum toxin is used in the treatment of dystonia: (*True/False*)

a the onset of effect is likely to occur within 24 h

b the effect is permanent

c it may be useful for spasm related to repetitive strain due to occupation

d it may be useful for spasm of facial, neck, eye and sphincter muscles.

BMJ. **303**: 40

BMJ. **305**: 1169–70

BMJ. **309**: 1526–7 (editorial)

4 A patient is making a steady recovery from what appears to be a typical attack of optic neuritis. On questioning she tells you that 2 years ago she noted numbness and tingling in her arm for a few weeks but did not bring it to a doctor's attention. She appears to have no suspicion of the implications of these problems. She has a happy marriage and a young family, and her husband is in stable employment. What are the advantages and disadvantages of referring her for a neurological opinion? Would you in fact refer her? (*5 points*)

BMJ. **309**: 392–5, 744

5 Multiple sclerosis.

a What proportion of sufferers experience at least one episode of major depression?

b What proportion of sufferers are likely to commit suicide?

BMJ. **315**: 691–2 (leading article)

6 Reflex sympathetic dystrophy. (*True/False*)

a Programmes of exercise, cryotherapy and galvanic stimulation have been demonstrated to be effective in controlled trials.

b Sympathetic blockade with guanethidine or bretylinum has been shown to be effective in long-term controlled trials.

BMJ. **310**: 1645–9

Parkinson's disease

1 The following support a diagnosis of Parkinson's disease: (*True/False*)

a coexisting seborrhoeic dermatitis

b more than one affected relative

c strictly unilateral symptoms for more than 3 years.

Br J Gen Pract. **45**: 261–6

2 What neurological syndromes are typified by the following clinical descriptions? (*5 points*)

a For several years an elderly man has had a coarse tremor of the hands and neck at rest. His voice is also unsteady. The problem is more marked when he is tense and if he has to hold his hand in a fixed position. There is cogwheel rigidity when you flex his elbow while he relaxes. There are no other abnormalities of motor function on examination.

b An elderly man walks with short steps and a broad-based gait. He holds on to grab rails and sometimes hesitates before initiating a step. Otherwise his movements are well co-ordinated and passive flexion of his joints is normal.

c An elderly man has noted progressive onset of stiffness and slowing of movements in his right arm. It now also affects his right leg. He is beginning to be unsteady on his legs and hesitates before starting to walk across the room. His facial expression is blank and his speech is slow. His writing is cramped and untidy. He has difficulty with finger-tapping exercises and with alternating supination and pronation of the wrist. His tendon reflexes are slightly brisker on the right side. When you flex his relaxed elbow you note initial resistance followed by cogwheel rigidity.

d A patient diagnosed as having Parkinson's disease while in his fifties has postural hypotension and urinary incontinence. Laevodopa-based treatment does not help him much, and it seems to bring on involuntary movements. His speech is slurred and quivering.

e A patient in his sixties has had frequent falls, usually falling backwards. His shirt front is smeared with food from his recent lunch. He notes difficulty in swallowing, and cannot pronounce words clearly. He holds his neck stiffly but needs to bend his head back when he wants to close his eyes.

BMJ. **310**: 447–52

3 Most patients with Parkinson's disease suffer from anosmia. (*True/False*)

BMJ. **310**: 1668

4 Patients with Parkinson's disease are usually overweight. (*True/False*)

BMJ. **301**: 256

5 What might be a useful way to test whether a patient with Parkinson's disease is fit to drive?

BMJ. **316**: 948 (citation)

6 Treatment of Parkinson's disease with levodopa. (*True/False*)

a Levodopa may cause postural hypotension.

b The introduction of levodopa should be delayed in patients with a long life-expectancy.

c The bioavailability of levodopa is affected by concurrent ingestion of protein.

d Domperidone is a useful treatment for nausea caused by levodopa.

BMJ. **310**: 575–9

7 In the treatment of Parkinson's disease: (*True/False*)

a patients on levodopa-based treatment have been shown to derive further benefit from the addition of selegiline

b bromocriptine is less effective than levodopa-based treatment

c bromocriptine is less likely than levodopa-based treatment to induce dyskinesias.

BMJ. **307**: 469–72

8 Metoclopramide is likely to exacerbate symptoms of Parkinson's disease. (*True/False*)

BMJ. **315**: 1096–9 (education and debate)

9 Subcutaneous apomorphine in Parkinson's disease.

a What are the potential benefits? (*3 points*)

b What preliminaries and procedures are needed when it is introduced? (*4 points*)

BMJ. **316**: 641 (leading article)

10 What health problems are more common in Parkinsonian patients who receive selegiline in addition to levodopa than in controls? (*2 points*)

BMJ. **316**: 1191–5

11 What surgical treatment could be offered for the following features of Parkinson's disease?

a Drug-resistant unilateral tremor.

b Akinesia or dyskinesia.

BMJ. **316**: 1259–60 (leading article)

ANSWERS

Diagnosis

1 Fundal examination for papilloedema. Observe heel-to-toe walking, which is sensitive to the effects of a posterior fossa tumour. Also cranial nerve palsies and persistent headache, worse on waking.

2 False.

3 Previously stable personality, nocturnal onset, little or no provocation, dramatic onset and offset, prominent motor features, repetitive or stereotyped behaviour, hallucinatory component, postictal confusion, family history of epilepsy, history of brain injury.

4 With neck pain, and pain and sensory disturbance in an upper limb. Usually sense of pain and temperature is lost but touch is preserved.

5 a Patient supine, with head tilted back 30 degrees and rotated 30 degrees to one side.
  b 6 months.
  c Habituation training – moving the head to the position that provokes the condition.

6 Gait disturbance, incontinence and mental deterioration.

7 False – it is probably due to primary orthostatic tremor.

8 Check for herpes zoster vesicles on the palate and the auditory meatus.

9 Round-ended needles push the fibres of dura mater aside rather than splitting them. Thus they reduce CSF leakage and the incidence of headache. For a similar reason the needles should be no wider than 22 gauge.

10 a True.
   b False.
   c False.

11 Presenting features are usually severe depression and/or disaesthesiae and paraesthesia, followed after several months by dementia, cerebellar signs, myoclonus and finally akinetic mutism.

12 Raised vibration threshold, particularly in the distribution of the median nerve.

13 a Myokymia, myotonia, epilepsy, possibly migraine.
   b Weakness, numbness.

14 a False – catecholamines and their metabolites are present in lower concentration in venous blood from affected limbs than from unaffected ones.
   b True – often in a spotty pattern.

Management

1 Clinical signs and symptoms are back pain, root pain, tingling, numbess and bladder dysfunction. If some or all of these are progressive, or if there is a history suggestive of cancer, immediate admission is warranted. Early surgical decompression greatly improves the prognosis.

2 Catheter gastrostomy.

3 a False – onset occurs within 1–4 days.

   b False – the first dose usually wears off in 1–15 weeks.

   c True.

   d True.

4 A patient in the prime of life and with a high level of responsibility develops symptoms that are likely to be due to demyelination, but she has not stated whether she suspects that she has a serious disorder.

   In deciding whether to refer her to a neurologist for formal diagnosis, doctors who addressed this question were conscious of the implications this would have for her expectations in life, her self-esteem and mood, and her career prospects and insurance premiums. The stress of undergoing investigation is a deterrent. Thereafter there is the prospect that she might adopt more of a sick role than would otherwise be the case, or that she would expose herself to false hopes of cure by expensive or troublesome treatments that have little proven efficacy.

   On the other hand, a gadolinium-enhanced MRI scan might show normal white matter, in which case her chances of having recurrent demyelination at 5 years are less than 3%. There is the prospect of reduced frequency of recurrences from treatment with interferon, and early use of steroids during exacerbations may limit their severity. If a positive diagnosis of MS is made, the woman would be able to decide whether further child-bearing was appropriate, and to make better plans for her career and the family finances. Early counselling, and also contact with the MS Society, may provide reassurance that the average prognosis is better than most people imagine.

   Most members therefore concluded that it would be paternalistic not to at least open the discussion of the prognosis with this woman, and gradually to introduce the possibility that this may be a recurring problem, and suggest that she might wish to have a better estimate of how likely this problem is to recur – without necessarily mentioning MS by its emotive name. The decision as to whether to refer for investigation can then be made in the light of the woman's own views and attitudes.

5 a 50%.

   b 1% in a study in Denmark and 15% in a 16-year follow-up study in Canada.

6 a False – the authors of a study comparing exercises and cryotherapy with and without galvanic stimulation reported benefit in both groups, but no placebo-controlled trials have been reported.

b False – in a trial comparing these treatments with lignocaine injection alone the authors found only a small minority of responders to either treatment.

Parkinson's disease

1 a True.
   b False – this suggests an alternative diagnosis.
   c False – this suggests cerebrovascular disease.

2 a Benign essential tremor.
   b Arteriosclerotic pseudoparkinsonism.
   c Parkinson's disease.
   d Shy Drager syndrome.
   e Steele Richardson Olszewski syndrome.

3 True – about 70% of patients with Parkinson's disease have anosmia, and about half of them are aware of it, so it is as common as tremor.

4 False – they are often underweight, possibly because tremor and hypertonia increase energy consumption, while bradykinesia and depression reduce food intake.

5 An on-the-road test is recommended. Perhaps a reaction timer would be a convenient screening guide.

6 a True.
   b True.
   c True.
   d True.

7 a False.
   b True.
   c True.

8 True.

9 a It overcomes refractory on-off periods and dyskinesias in patients who are resistant to levodopa. It reduces levodopa-induced nausea, and has a lower incidence of neuropsychiatric complications than other oral anti-Parkinsonian agents.
   b Counselling, pretreatment with domperidone for 3 days, ECG to rule out cardiac arrhythmia, and then a challenge dose to establish whether a response occurs and to define the appropriate dose.

10 Falls and dementia.

11 a Unilateral thalamotomy or a thalamic stimulator.
    b Pallidotomy.

PAEDIATRICS

Accidents

1 What non-surgical measure may help a child to expel a foreign body trapped in a nostril? (*1 point*)

BMJ. **312**: 1620 (citation)

2 Why might a child put superglue on his eyelids? (*1 point*)

BMJ. **313**: 124 (brief report)

3 A toddler has sucked the spout of a teapot containing freshly made tea. He does not appear distressed 30 min later. What dangers may lie in store? (*2 points*)

BMJ. **307**:923

4 A mother rings to say that she spilt talcum powder on her baby's face during a nappy change. She can be reassured that this is unlikely to cause a problem. (*True/False*)

BMJ. **302**: 1200–1

5 A child who has swallowed a coin should have his abdomen X-rayed. (*True/False*)

BMJ. **302**: 1321–2

6 Swallowed objects.

a Injection of what drug may relax the cardiac sphincter sufficiently to relieve oesophagospasm or allow a swallowed coin to pass into the stomach?

b What sort of swallowed foreign body is best retrieved even if it has passed into the stomach?

BMJ. **302**: 1607

7 The parents of a child with an unexplained fracture say that the child 'must have brittle bones'. List four or more findings on history or physical examination that would support this contention.

BMJ. **302**: 1244

Urogenital system

1 Phimosis.

a What proportion of foreskins retract partially at birth?

b What proportion of foreskins retract at the age of 5 years?

c What proportion of foreskins retract at the age of 17 years?

BMJ. **306**: 1-2

2 Urogenital surgery.

a What simple procedure can treat phimosis in a male toddler? (*1 point*)

b At what age is hypospadias usually treated surgically? (*1 point*)

*BMJ.***12**: 299–301 (review article)

3 What dosage form of antibiotic is particularly suitable for treating infections under the prepuce in a small boy?

BMJ. **312**: 1230

4 Behaviour and emotions are more important than genetic influences in the aetiology of enuresis. (*True/False*)

BMJ. **302**: 729

5 In the management of an enuretic child aged 8 years:

a what approaches can the child and his parents use to control the problem without resorting to drugs or equipment? (*3 points*)

b what apparatus should be provided? (*2 points*)

c which drug is likely to be most helpful? (*1 point*)

BMJ. **306**: 536,1003

6 What is your policy on collecting and examining urine samples from infants with feverish illnesses or vomiting but no localizing features? (*4 points*)

BMJ. **307**: 761–4, 1141–2

7 When using urine collection pads for obtaining samples from infants or the incontinent confused elderly, what instructions should be given to the supervisor?

Br J Gen Pract. **48**: 1342–3 (letter)

8 Pyuria in a child is diagnostic of a urinary tract infection. (*True/False*)

BMJ. **311**:924 (original article)

9 A 3-year-old has had a single proven episode of urinary infection with fever and vomiting. What radiological investigation should you request?

BMJ. **304**: 663–5

10 After reaching what age does a child with a history of UTI appear to have negligible risk of acquiring a renal scar demonstrable on DMSA scan?

BMJ. **315**: 905–8 (research report)

11 Suprapubic aspiration is a suitable procedure for the GP surgery. Do you agree with this? State reasons for your point of view. If you agree with the statement, describe what preliminaries you would undertake before the procedure.

BMJ. **309**: 1042

ENT and respiratory system

1 What mechanisms may cause blockage of the Eustachian tube in a baby?
Br J Gen Pract. **41**: 258

2 Good advice for parents of a 3-month-old baby with catarrh include the following. (*True/False*)

a The baby should sleep with a pillow.

b The baby should sleep on his back rather than on his side or his front.

c An apnoea alarm will indicate if the baby's airway is obstructed.

d Having the baby in the parents' room may reduce the risk of sudden death.

e It is important to wrap the baby up tightly in the cot.

f The baby's feet should be near the footboard of the cot.

Br J Gen Pract. **41**: 431

3 What better alternative to an apnoea monitor is now available for monitoring infants who are at high risk of sudden infant death syndrome?

BMJ. **304**: 266

4 Which infants are at increased risk of sudden infant death syndrome? What can be done about this in infants who are discovered to be at risk?

BMJ. **316**: 1852 (news item), 179–80

5 Infantile bronchiolitis: (*True/False*)

a can sometimes be differentiated from asthma by the presence of crackles

b is spread by aerosol droplets

c is likely to respond to nebulized salbutamol

d is likely to respond to steroids.

BMJ. **310**: 4–5 (editorial)

6 The following factors in a child with otitis media are associated with fever and earache lasting a further 3 days or more:

a onset in winter

b age under 2 years.

BMJ. **303**: 1450–2

7 What benefits and drawbacks can be expected from prescribing antibiotics (mainly amoxycillin, ampicillin or penicillin in this meta-analysis) for children with otitis media?

BMJ. **314**: 1526–9 (meta-analysis)

8 How may breathing rates be demonstrated to mothers who need to be able to recognize tachypnoea in a baby?

BMJ. **304**: 637

9 Oral dexamethasone, 0.15 mg/kg, for croup has been shown in a placebo-controlled trial to have the following benefits. (*True/False*)

a It reduces demand for further medical attention.

b It reduces the duration of symptoms.

BMJ. **313**: 140–2

10 How soon after administering nebulized steroid to a child with croup can benefit be expected?

BMJ. **311**: 1244 (editorial)

Gastrointestinal system

1 If in doubt after a clinical examination, what is the investigation of choice to establish whether an infant has pyloric stenosis?

BMJ. **312**: 236–9

2 How would you advise the mother of an infant with diarrhoea if she requests information on how to make up her own sugar and electrolyte solution as she has no access to a pharmacy? (*3 points*)

BMJ. **305**: 1111-12

3 Cows' milk protein intolerance. (*True/False*)

a A history of chronic diarrhoea, fretful behaviour and a rash on introduction of cows' milk is sufficient for a diagnosis.

b Soya milk is the ideal treatment.

BMJ. **313**: 507 (leading article)

4 What initial investigation would be appropriate for a 6-month-old infant who has had diarrhoea for 4 weeks and in whom stool cultures have been negative?

BMJ. **302**: 545–6

5 If treating a child with diarrhoea with a soya-based milk: (*True/False*)

a the treatment should be continued until the child is 4 years old

b lactose in the soya-based milk may cause continued diarrhoea

c the infant's height and weight should be measured regularly

d a calcium supplement is required

e a vitamin D supplement may be beneficial.

BMJ. **303**: 177

6 What clinical features would lead you to suspect intussusception in an infant or young child?

BMJ. **304**: 737–9

7 What investigation would be appropriate for a child who has had constipation for as long as his mother can remember?

BMJ. **305**: 462–4

Nervous system

1 You are called to see a 15-month-old child at home as an emergency because he has had a fever for 2 days and a fit lasting 10 min in the past hour. The parents blame the MMR injection that the child received 5 days ago.

a What information will you need to obtain to help you decide whether to request hospital admission?

b You decide that the child may stay at home. What advice do you give the parents?

BMJ. **303**: 634–5

Growth

1 From what organization can one obtain sets of UK child growth charts extending to the 0.4th centile (3 standard deviations from the mean)?

BMJ. **308**: 641–2

2 Measuring children's growth.

a What set of charts can be used to compare the rate of a child's weight gain over a given time period with population reference values?

b What chart can be used to determine whether a child is unusually fat or thin for his or her age?

c On what population were these charts of reference values based?

BMJ. **311**: 583 (leader)

3 What are the limitations of the following indices of growth when assessing a child's general health?

- Height.
- Height velocity over 6 months.

BMJ. **305**: 1400–2
BMJ. **306**: 270–1

4 Failure to thrive in childhood affects weight for age before it affects height for age. (*True/False*)

BMJ. **308**: 596

5 What proportion of children below the fifth centile for height at age 7 years can be expected to remain below the fifth centile at the age of 23 years?

BMJ. **310**: 696–9

6 When considering whether a short child will benefit from growth-hormone treatment: (*True/False*)

a a short child who has grown less than 4 cm in the past year requires an explanation

b the effect of long-term growth-hormone treatment on final height is predictable

c daily injections are required

d growth-hormone treatment involves risks that necessitate regular follow-up at a specialist centre.

BMJ. **304**: 131–2

7 What laboratory tests are indicated for a 5-year-old child at or below the third percentile for height for no readily explicable reason? (*3 points*)

BMJ. **305**:1400–2

8 A short 15-year-old with delayed development of secondary sexual characteristics has been investigated and no evidence of endocrine tumour or hyperplasia has been identified. What other risks are there for this adolescent?

BMJ. **305**:790

Hereditary conditions

1 The parents of a child with a rare inherited condition which will necessitate long and close support would like to know more about the experience of families with a similar problem. What organization may provide this information for them?

BMJ. **303**: 1154

2 In the detection and management of congenital dislocation of the hip: (*True/ False*)

   a most hips found to be unstable on day 1 will be normal on re-examination a week later

   b early splinting is free of any dangers

   c repeated clinical examination is harmless

   d X-ray provides a reliable diagnosis in the neonate

   e the prevalence of CDH is about 1 in 500 births.

BMJ. **305**: 435, 521

3 What is the investigation of choice in an infant with suspected congenital dislocation of the hip?

BMJ. **310**: 917–19

4 What are the advantages of identifying babies with Duchenne muscular dystrophy as soon as they are born when there is no effective treatment? (*2 points*)

BMJ. **306**: 349

5 The following clinical features would raise a suspicion of cystic fibrosis in a baby: (*True/False*)

   a prolonged jaundice

   b recurrent vomiting

   c nasal polyps

   d the infant becoming floppy in warm weather

   e tetany.

BMJ. **308**: 459–61

Miscellaneous

1 Putting sugar solution in the mouth of a neonate immediately before lancing the heel reduces the duration of crying. (*True/False*)

BMJ. **310**: 1498–50

2 Sticky eye in infancy.

   a What clinical features would suggest a diagnosis of congenital lacrimal obstruction? (*5 points*)

b What clinical features would suggest a diagnosis more serious than congenital lacrimal obstruction? (*5 points*)

BMJ. **315**: 293–6 (review)

3 In a child suffering recurrent infections, what findings on history or physical examination would suggest that testing for hypogammaglobulinaemia is indicated? (*3 points*)

BMJ. **308**: 581–5

4 Younger children in large families suffer more atopic disease than their older siblings. (*True/False*)

BMJ. **308**: 692–4

5 What is now the official advice on how to minimize sensitization of infants to peanut?

BMJ. **316**: 1926 (news item)

6 Is a GP wise to provide a booklet of advice to mothers on:

a treatment of their childrens' ailments

b circumstances when an emergency visit by the GP is justifiable?

Give two reasons for your point of view in each case.

BMJ. **303**: 1111-14

7 A baby has thrush on his perineum. What is the probability that he also has thrush in his mouth?

Br J Gen Pract. **42**: 490–1

8 According to the current state of knowledge, which children may justify screening for insulin antibodies? (*2 points*)

BMJ. **307**:1435–6

9 A teenage boy develops gynaecomastia. What is the prognosis? (*1 point*)

BMJ. **309**: 797–800

10 Flat red horizontal streaks on the skin over the lumbar area in an adolescent are probably due to injury. (*True/False*)

BMJ. **311**: 738 (original article)

ANSWERS

Accidents

1 Nebulized adrenalin reduces mucosal swelling, loosens the foreign body and may make it possible to expel it by exhaling with the other nostril closed off.

2 He might mistake it for a tube of ophthalmic antibiotic ointment.

3 Swelling of the epiglottis and peritonsillar area causing blockage of the airway.

4 False – talcum powder contains magnesium silicate, a potent irritant to the airways. There are 30 reports in the literature of it leading to serious respiratory problems requiring hospital attention and causing 8 deaths.

5 False – only a chest X-ray is required, as any obstacle to the passage of the coin will be at the cardiac sphincter.

6 a Glucagon.
  b A battery.

7 History of recurrent fractures in one parent, history of recurrent fractures while in foster care, finding of blue sclerae, dentinogenesis imperfecta or hypermobile joints.

Urogenital system

1 a 50%.
  b 90%.
  c 99%.

2 a Preputial stretch under local anaesthesia, e.g. with Emla cream.
  b The second or third year of life.

3 Eye ointment is supplied with a convenient nozzle for applying it.

4 False – in most cases one can obtain a history of enuresis in emotionally stable first-degree relatives.

5 a Hygiene, bladder exercises, avoiding a punitive parental attitude, contacting the Enuresis Resource and Information Centre.
  b A star chart and an enuresis alarm.
  c Desmopressin – for short-term use, e.g. when sleeping away from home.

6 We all recognize the importance of diagnosing urine infections in fevered babies and toddlers, but the history and examination may provide no clues. Several GPs

addressing this problem felt anxious about the difficulties that this posed. Mothers should perhaps be encouraged to have a fresh urine sample available for the doctor at the consultation if their child has a fever but no chest symptoms or catarrh. A fresh potty sample will suffice. Sitting a child on a cold surface often provokes micturition. For babies in nappies a cotton-wool pad can be placed inside the nappy and wrung into the specimen container, which should then be stored in a refrigerator. This is advice that might be included in the practice leaflet and given by receptionists to mothers who request a home visit. Some practices make perineal pouch collection bags available to mothers on request. Several members mentioned that they carry Multistix and universal containers in their bags to test for protein, red cells, nitrite and leucocyte esterase.

7 Pads should be checked every 10 to 20 min in babies. The urine is withdrawn with a syringe, and can be placed in a universal container which is kept in a refrigerator. The pads are available from NHS stores (Order No. CFQ 152).

8 False – moderate pyuria (10–100×10^6 leucocytes/L) was found in 43% of feverish children and 6% of afebrile children, and obvious pyuria (100–700×10^6 leucocytes/L) in 9% of feverish children in this survey.

9 Ultrasound is a simple, non-invasive technique, which may be used to demonstrate reflux. A DMSA scintiscan is the best technique for demonstrating renal scarring.

10 4 years of age.

11 If the bladder of neonates is found to contain urine on ultrasound examination the procedure is 100% successful, but without prior scanning the success rate is only 36%. In view of the trauma of the procedure, it is best performed under ultrasound control.

ENT and respiratory system

1 Infection, atopy and gastric reflux.

2 a False.
   b True.
   c False.
   d True.
   e False – bedclothes should be sufficiently tight to prevent the baby from slipping under them, but no tighter than this.
   f True – this reduces the risk that the baby will slip under the bedclothes.

3 Percutaneous monitoring of oxygen saturation.

4 Almost half of 24 infants who died suddenly, mainly in the second or third month of life, were found to have had a prolonged QT interval recorded on ECG at birth. The upper limit of normal for QT interval in neonates is 440 ms, and this identified 12 of the 24 deaths. Obstructive apnoea is more common in infants who later die suddenly.

An increased incidence of sudden infant death syndrome is reported in the families of patients with obstructive sleep apnoea. There has been one report that retroposition of the maxilla and mandible is common in both conditions.

Beta-blockers might prevent arrhythmias. However, there was no familial association in these cases. The 24 cases were from a study group of 100 000, and 100 individuals might require treatment to prevent two deaths.

5 a True.

    b False – nasal secretions spread by hand contact or fomites.

    c True.

    d False.

6 a False.

    b True.

7 Benefits and drawbacks include the following:
- no difference in continuing pain at 24 h (typically about 65% recover within 24 h)
- a 41% reduction in pain scores at 2–7 days
- a reduction in tympanic perforations from about 8% to about 4%
- increased risk of vomiting, diarrhoea or rash from about 11% to about 16%
- no difference in abnormalities on tympanometry at 1 month at about 35%
- reduction in contralateral acute otitis media from about 17% to about 9%
- no difference in the incidence of recurrence at about 22%.

8 With a string-and-weight pendulum:
2 m length = 21 breaths/min
1 m length = 30 breaths/min
35 cm length = 50 breaths/min.

9 a True.

    b False.

10 Within 2–4 h.

Gastrointestinal system

1 Ultrasound examination.

2 Before advising a parent on how to make up a rehydration solution, members thought it worth finding out whether the chemist might be able to deliver the sachets, or else the doctor could provide some from his or her bag. Several members were reluctant to advise a parent to make up a solution. Perhaps one should only give the following advice to particularly able parents.

One litre of most rehydration solutions contains about 100 mmol of glucose and 60 mmol of sodium, partly as chloride and partly as bicarbonate. A level teaspoonful of table salt weighs about 4 g and provides approximately 70 mmol of sodium. A level teaspoonful of baking soda also weighs about 4 g and provides about 50 mmol of sodium as bicarbonate. A level tablespoonful of granulated sugar weighs approximately 20 g, representing about 55 mmol of sucrose. After the action of disaccharidase, this will provide 55 mmol of glucose and 55 mmol of fructose in the gut lumen. Thus a reasonable solution could be made up with a level tablespoonful of sugar or 50 mL of concentrated fruit squash (about 40% sugar) and a level teaspoonful of salt in 1 L of water. It would be better to use glucose instead of sugar. A half teaspoonful of bicarbonate and a half teaspoonful of salt rather than a whole teaspoonful of salt would be a further refinement. Potassium may be provided from dried fruit or bananas, as soon as the child can face these.

3 a False – a more exhaustive investigation is needed.

   b False – protein hydrolysate would be better, as soya is also a potential allergen.

4 Colonoscopy as the first investigation. Chronic infantile diarrhoea is commonly due to bacterial infection, Crohn's disease, coeliac disease, necrotizing enterocolitis, or allergy to cow's milk or soya milk.

5 a False – most diarrhoea due to cow's-milk protein intolerance abates by the age of 18–36 months, and a challenge test at about this age should be performed.

   b False – soya products are useful for lactose intolerance.

   c True.

   d False – provided that infant-formula soya milk is used, which contains supplementary calcium.

   e True – an additional 7–10 mcg of vitamin D per day should be given as the dose in the infant formula soya milk is insufficient.

6 Vomiting (especially if bilious), abdominal pain, rectal bleeding (the classical redcurrant-jelly stool), abdominal mass, fever and lethargy.

7 A barium enema on an unprepared bowel, with a film 24 h later, is sometimes used as a screening investigation. Manometry and rectal biopsy will also be required to confirm a diagnosis of Hirschsprung's disease.

Nervous system

1 a The following information is needed.
   - Is it a first fit?
   - Description of the fit – assess its duration, whether it was focal, and time to recovery of consciousness.
   - Past history of neurological problems.
   - Family history of convulsions.
   - Degree of parental ability and anxiety.

- Availability for follow-up.
- Infant's muscle tension.
- Infant's co-ordination and level of response.
- Infant's ocular reflexes.
- Presence of a rash.
- Kernig and Brudzinsky signs.
- Blood glucose if the infant is poorly rousable.

b Several GP respondents favoured sending the child to hospital purely on the basis of the information provided in the question.

Among those GPs who were willing to let the child stay at home, answers included the following.

i Prognosis:

- benign in later childhood and adulthood
- likelihood of recurrence during fever lessens after the age of 3–4 years
- use of paracetamol, ibuprofen, tepid sponging and cool drinks during fever
- use of rectal diazepam if a fit occurs.

ii Explain that MMR vaccine may cause fever in a minority of those who receive it, and that it may have been a factor in precipitating this convulsion. However, it is no more likely than other causes of fever to bring about a convulsion, and if the child fell ill with any of the illnesses that MM prevents, he would be even more likely to have a fever.

iii Make sure that the family has a thermometer and knows how to use it.

iv Call the doctor if the fever worsens or if fitting recurs.

Growth

1 The Child Growth Foundation, 2 Mayfield Avenue, London W4 1PW.

2 a Conditional reference charts.
   b Children's body mass index charts.
   c White children between 1978 and 1990.

3 A child may be short compared to his or her parents at the same age because of a current chronic medical or emotional problem, or because a previous illness has not yet been followed by sufficient catch-up growth. A series of height readings therefore provides better guidance than a single reading. However, growth of an individual child proceeds at a varying pace, and 2 years may be required for an adequate assessment of growth rate. Growth rate measurements are subject to the combined errors of the individual height observations, and complete reliance on them may lead to undue delay in investigating a growth problem.

4 True.

5 29–31%.

6 a True.

b False.

c True.

d False – there are no specific dangers.

7 Full blood count, thyroid function, then perhaps urinary growth hormone. Jejunal biopsy and sweat test might be considered if the history suggests coeliac disease or cystic fibrosis.

8 Social ostracism leading to impaired mental health. Osteoporosis. Disproportionate limbs.

Hereditary conditions

1 Contact a Family, 16 Strutton Ground, London SW1P 2HP.

2 a True.

b False.

c False.

d False.

e True.

3 Dynamic ultrasound.

4 Earlier diagnosis permits genetic counselling and prenatal diagnosis in future pregnancies.

5 a True.

b False.

c True.

d True.

e False.

Miscellaneous

1 True – this author found that mean crying time in the first 3 min after the procedure decreased from 130 s in controls to 50 s in those given 2 mL of 50% sucrose solution.

2 a Epiphora, crusting, clear cornea, pressure at the inner canthus expressing mucopus from the canaliculi, failure of a drop of fluorescein to clear from the eye within 5 min.

    b • Persistent rubbing, red eye, photophobia, systemic upset, proptosis or impaired vision, suggesting conjunctivitis, keratitis or congenital glaucoma.

      • A skin fold at the lid margin pushing the lashes into the conjunctiva (congenital epiblepharon).

      • Hyperaemia of the lower fornix, suggesting chlamydial infection.

3 Failure to thrive, congenital absence of tonsils, hepatosplenomegaly, arthropathy.

4 False – the firstborn is more likely to be atopic than younger siblings.

5 Pregnant mothers with a history of atopy should not eat peanut. Children from families with a history of allergy should avoid peanut until the age of 3 years. In any case all children should avoid whole peanuts until the age of 5 years to prevent the risk of choking.

6 Doctors who provided written information for mothers on how to cope with children's ailments have reported that it reduced the number of surgery consultations, but only at the cost of an increased number of out-of-hours visits when the need for reassurance was more than could be met by printed information. GPs addressing this question felt that these leaflets would be appreciated by families bringing up their first child in the absence of grandparents. However, it can be difficult to present information for people with limited reading ability. It could be helpful to provide a list of useful home remedies for mothers to keep in stock. Given the wide variability in illnesses, circumstances, and mothers' attitudes and abilities, it would be particularly difficult to present details of circumstances in which it is appropriate to call the doctor. If such a leaflet is used it may be helpful to discuss the text with the mother during a consultation. It might be better to mention the availability of a doctor for telephone advice, rather than to suggest that mothers request visits in the first instance.

7 About 60% from the results of this study.

8 Possibly those with one or more relatives with insulin-dependent diabetes and who have been bottle fed.

9 80% of cases resolve spontaneously within 2 years.

10 False – these are probably physiological striae due to rapid growth.

RENAL DISEASE

1 What percentage of the population is carrying organ donor cards?

BMJ. **306**: 869

2 What is the significance of finding the following types of cast on microscopy of urine?

a Hyaline.

b Casts containing red cells.

c Casts containing other types of cells.

BMJ. **312**: 1090–4 (review)

3 A raised serum urea concentration in the presence of an unchanged serum creatinine concentration may be due to: (*True/False*)

a physical exercise

b fever

c early bilateral urinary obstruction

d dehydration

e congestive cardiac failure.

BMJ. **302**: 651

4 Urine for protein output has usually been collected over 24 h. What advantages and pitfalls are there in making an alternative measurement of the ratio of urine protein to creatinine in a spot urine sample?

BMJ. **316**: 504–9 (research report)

5 A high intake of what fluid may increase the risk of kidney stones?

BMJ. **316**: 1326 (citation)

6 Which patients with renal colic should be admitted to hospital? (*3 or more points*)

BMJ. **312**: 132 (citation)

7 Alfacalcidol supplements for 2 years in mild to moderate renal failure: (*True/False*)

   a can cause a temporary reduction in parathyroid hormone levels

   b have been shown to reduce fracture rates

   c have been shown to reduce bone pain

   d improve bone histology if there are pre-existing features of renal osteody-strophy

   e need to have the dose monitored by regular measurements of serum calcium.

   BMJ. **310**: 358–63

8 In chronic renal failure: (*True/False*)

   a hyperparathyroidism may contribute to causing the anaemia

   b ferritin is useless as a measure of iron stores

   c aluminium toxicity may cause a microcytic anaemia

   d the ESR is useless as an index of acute inflammation.

   BMJ. **310**: 1424–5

9 Managing chronic renal failure.

   a What form of dyslipidaemia is most common?

   b What cautions are needed when prescribing lipid-lowering agents? (*2 points*)

   c What seems to be the most practical measure when checking for iron deficiency?

   d What seem to be the most practical measures when checking for nutritional deficiency?

   e i What serum abnormality tends to bring on secondary hyperparathyroidism?

   ii How may secondary hyperparathyroidism be prevented? (*3 points*)

   BMJ. **315**: 1429–32 (review).

10 Apart from raising the haemoglobin level, what other physiological benefits do patients with chronic renal failure derive from erythropoietin?

   BMJ. **316**: 1178 (citation)

ANSWERS

1 18%.

2 a No clinical importance.

   b Suggests glomerulonephritis.

   c Indicates tubular damage.

3 a False.

   b True.

   c True.

   d True.

   e True.

4 Albuminuria is increased by erect posture, strenuous exercise, hot or cold tempera-tures, intercurrent illness and fever. Creatinine excretion varies directly with muscle mass.

   The advantages of measuring the ratio of albumin to creatinine in a spot sample are as follows:

   • sample collection is much easier

   • samples are more reliable, as some 24-h collections are likely to be incomplete

   • a spot sample collected first thing in the morning will have been formed when the patient was supine, and will thus be free of the effect of posture and exercise. The disadvantages of using the ratio are as follows:

   • it will be affected by the errors in both assays

   • muscle mass affecting creatinine excretion may influence interpretation of the assay. Reference ranges for the ratio are different for men and women

   • physical training may reduce the ratio merely by increasing muscle mass.

5 Grapefruit juice.

6 Those with intractable pain and those with evidence of systemic upset suggestive of associated pyelonephritis, i.e. fever, vomiting.

7 a True.

   b False.

   c True.

   d True.

   e True.

8 a True – it causes marrow fibrosis.

   b False – but liver disease, acute inflammation and malignancy do render ferritin useless, as it is an acute-phase protein.

   c True.

    d True.

9 **a** Raised triglyceride.

    b • Fibrates are used in low dose as there is a risk of myositis and rhabdomyolysis.

       • Interaction between cyclosporin and HMG CoA reductase inhibitors.

    c The percentage of hypochromic cells is likely to be less than 10% in the absence of iron deficiency.

    d Weight loss, serum albumin.

    e i Raised serum phosphate.

       ii Controlled dietary intake of protein, 0.8–1.0 g/kg/day.

       • Calcium carbonate or acetate, 1.5 g with meals.

       • Oral supplements of vitamin D_3 once the serum phosphate is controlled.

10 Improved nutritional status, reflected in raised serum albumin levels and body weight.

RESPIRATORY DISEASE

Diagnosis

1 What are the five commonest organisms cultured from elderly patients with community acquired pneumonia?

BMJ. **316**: 1690 (leading article)

2 In obstructive airways disease, the need for long-term oxygen treatment can be rationally assessed on the basis of three measurements. What are they?

Drug Ther Bull. **28**: 99–100

3 In obstructive airways disease, the FEV_1 is more likely to decline with the passing years than is the peak flow rate. (*True/False*)

Br J Gen Pract. **45**: 15–18 (research report)

4 Reduced FEV_1 is a risk factor for death from stroke. List or devise three hypotheses that might explain this finding.

BMJ. **302**:8447

5 What life-style factor appears to be associated with the presence of oedema in patients with chronic bronchitis?

BMJ. **306**: 374

6 How do patients with Wegener's granulomatosis present?

a List four or more common clinical features.

b Name a test that is valuable in reaching the diagnosis.

BMJ. **304**: 269

7 Wegener's granulomatosis: (*True/False*)

a commonly affects the gums

b causes renal failure

c is treatable.

BMJ. **309**: 111–12

Management

1 In treating the common cold, which remedies are supported by good evidence? (*6 points*)

BMJ. **316**: 33–6 (review)

2 You are writing an advice sheet for adult patients on treating common symptoms. Under what circumstances would you advise a patient with cough:

a to self-treat

b to consult the practice nurse

c to consult the doctor?

Br J Gen Pract. **41**: 289–92

3 The following are to be expected in adults with chronic obstructive airways disease on maintenance treatment with inhaled bronchodilators alone. (*True/False*)

a Over 1 year FEV_1 declines significantly more in patients treated four times per day with inhaled bronchodilators than in those treated intermittently on demand.

b The decline in FEV_1 is similar in patients with bronchitis and those with asthma.

c The decline is similar in patients treated with salbutamol and those treated with ipratropium bromide.

d Patients who are advised to use their inhalers on demand use them once a day on average.

e Patients who are on continuous treatment prefer salbutamol to ipratropium.

f Patients who are on intermittent on-demand treatment prefer salbutamol to ipratropium.

BMJ. **303** 1426–31

BMJ. **304**: 21

4 What benefits have been demonstrated from a programme of physical exercise for patients with chronic obstructive airways disease? (*4 or more points*)

BMJ. **314**: 1361 (leading article)

5 On the basis of current evidence, what appear to be the indications for non-invasive positive pressure ventilation for patients with acute exacerbations of obstructive pulmonary disease? (*3 or more points*)

BMJ. **314**: 163–4 (leading article)

6 What surgical procedure is of proven benefit for a patient with end-stage emphysema?

BMJ. **309**: 1244 (editorial)

7 How can you produce a flap valve over an intravenous cannula as emergency treatment of a tension pneumothorax?

BMJ. **311**:1506 (letter)

8 What measures should a pigeon fancier take to minimize exposure to inhaled avian antigens while continuing with his hobby? (*5 points*)

BMJ. **315**: 70–1

9 Current quantitative assays of antibodies causing pigeon fancier's lung or farmer's lung give reliable results. (*True/False*)

BMJ. **315**: 1311 (letter)

10 What discomforts associated with nose masks are likely to reduce patients' compliance with continuous positive airway pressure for sleep apnoea?

BMJ. **316**: 1470 (citation)

11 What nebulized drug is used to suppress cough due to lung cancer?

BMJ. **304**: 718

ANSWERS

Diagnosis

1 • *Streptococcus pneumoniae* (up to 40% of cases)
   • *Chlamydia pneumoniae* (up to 26% of cases)
   • *Mycoplasma pneumoniae* (3–23% of cases)
   • *Haemophilus influenzae* (5–8% of cases)
   • *Legionella pneumophila* (3–6% of cases)

2 • FEV_1 (less than 1.5 L)
   • PaO_2 (less than 7.3 kPa)
   • Peripheral oedema.
   This combination of indications was associated with improved survival after use of long-term oxygen treatment in clinical trials in the UK and America.

3 True.

4 • Chronic hypoxia leads to relative polycythaemia, which results in thrombosis.
   • Chronic hypercarbia leads to loss of respiratory drive and sleep apnoea, which promotes thrombosis.
   • Common precursors, e.g. alcohol, vitamin C deficiency, air pollution, hereditary predisposition, smoking (although this last factor was controlled for in the study).

5 High alcohol consumption.

6 a Chronic sinusitis, nosebleeds, painful red eyes, joint pains, sensory loss, fever and weight loss.
   b Antineutrophil cytoplasmic antibody.

7 a True.
   b True.
   c True – using steroids and cyclophosphamide.

Management

1 First-generation antihistamines and intranasal ipratropium reduce rhinorrhoea. Alpha-adrenergic agonists do so as well, but they carry a risk of rebound on discontinuation and hypertension. Inhaling steam, and using intranasal cromoglycate or nedocromil, will ease symptoms. Naproxen reduces headache, malaise and cough.
   Intranasal steroids are ineffective. The efficacy of vitamin C and zinc supplements is unproven. Antibiotics only help if bacteria are cultured from the nasal secretions.

Guaiaphenesin reduces sputum thickness and quantity and has a slight antitussive effect. Antiseptic solution (2% iodine in the trial) applied to volunteers' fingers reduced transmission rates.

2   The following is based on a consensus of answers from GPs.

    For fit adults with a single episode of cough, self-treatment is appropriate unless the cough lasts for more than a week or two, or is accompanied by breathlessness, severe or prolonged fever, chest pain, wheeze, or blood in the sputum. Frail elderly patients and babies require an earlier consultation with the doctor. If the purpose of the consultation is merely to obtain an NHS prescription for free linctus, the practice nurse might usefully ask questions to rule out a serious problem and then ask the GP to sign a prescription. However, in many practices the practice nurses are as heavily booked as the doctors.

3   **a** True. 0.72 L/year compared to 0.20 L/year.

    b True.

    c True.

    d False – median usage in this study was 0.3 inhalations per day.

    e False.

    f True – perhaps because of its faster onset of action.

4   Increased exercise capacity and physical endurance, better emotional function, feeling less breathless and feeling more in control of their illness.

5   Dyspnoea, raised respiratory rate, acidosis, hypoxia.

6   Single lung transplantation.

7   Pass the cannula through the finger of a sterile surgical glove from within. Insert the cannula into the pleural cavity and attach the glove around the junction of the cannula to its hub. The glove flops over the open end of the cannula to form a valve.

8   • Wear a well-fitting mask made to European Standard EN149 FFP2S.

    • Wear a coat and hat that are removed on leaving the pigeon loft.

    • Restrict time spent in the pigeon loft to a minimum.

    • Avoid scraping out or cleaning the loft.

    • Avoid transporting pigeons on the back seat of the car.

9   False.

10 The masks often leak and they are associated with a dry mouth and throat.

11 Lignocaine.

STROKE

1   Transient ischaemic attacks may sometimes be due to cerebral haemorrhage. (*True/False*)

BMJ. **316**: 1495–6 (case reports)

2   Blood pressure after a stroke. (*True/False*)
  a Blood pressure usually rises in the first few days after a stroke.
  b Low blood pressure immediately after a stroke requires treatment.
  c It is unwise to lower the diastolic blood pressure below 110 mmHg in the first few days after a stroke.
  d Lowering raised blood pressure in the long term after a stroke has been shown to reduce the probability of a recurrence.

BMJ. **308**: 1523–4

3   List two categories of stroke victim, other than those who require nursing care, for whom urgent admission to a neurological unit may be beneficial.

BMJ. **302**: 1565–7

4   If one of your patients with a reasonable quality of life had a stroke, would you want him or her to have a CT scan within a few days? Give reasons for your answer. (*3 or more points*)

BMJ. **309**:1498–50 (discussion papers)

5   Information in the history and clinical signs when a stroke patient is first seen will help to determine whether antithrombotic therapy is justified and whether a neurosurgical opinion is justified. What are the relevant observations? (*9 points*)

BMJ. **308**: 1674–6

6   What resources are needed for optimal rehabilitation of a patient with hemiparesis and dysarthria after a stroke? (*3 or more points*)

BMJ. **309**: 1356–8 (discussion paper)

7 Robert, aged 53 years, was working as a garage mechanic until a stroke paralysed his left side 2 months ago. He has now returned home from hospital to his two-storey semi-detached house and his wife, who has been dreading having to look after him. He was formerly a binge drinker and quite rude and insensitive to her after drinking. A helpful daughter lives a mile away with her young family. Robert is now quite pleasant and cheerful and looks a lot healthier for being debarred from alcohol and tobacco for 2 months. He needs help to chop his food, to rise from bed, to get to the upstairs bathroom and to get in and out of the bath. He is keen to become as mobile as possible and to drive a car again. The couple have major financial worries because the mortgage has not yet been paid off.

What matters might you discuss with this couple? What targets might you discuss as possibly appropriate for the next week before you call again, and for the next few months? (*7 or more points*)

BMJ. **313**: 677–81 (review)

8 Patients with inco-ordination of swallowing: (*True/False*)

a find it easier to swallow fluids than soft solids

b can be identified by an impaired gag reflex.

BMJ. **312**: 972–3 (correspondence)

9 Inserting a gastrostomy tube to feed a stroke victim with dysphagia: (*True/False*)

a improves survival

b requires a general anaesthetic.

BMJ. **312**: 13–15 (research article)

ANSWERS

1 True – case reports are presented.

2 a True.
  b True.
  c True.
  d False.

3 Patients with probable cerebral haemorrhages and patients with infarction due to embolism.

4 A CT scan in the first week after a stroke is currently the most widely available and reliable way to differentiate between cerebral haemorrhage and infarction, although it is likely to be superseded by MRI scans in the future. A CT scan may also lead to a positive diagnosis of the rare subdural haematoma or subarachnoid haemorrhage which require specific treatment, or an atypical presentation of tumour, abscess or (by exclusion) migraine. It costs less than a day of in-patient treatment. A positive diagnosis of infarction may lead to aspirin treatment and ultrasound studies of the carotids, as well as detailed cardiac observations looking for atrial fibrillation, SBE or myxoma. A positive diagnosis of cerebral haemorrhage may lead to lowering of the blood pressure being given higher priority and aspirin being avoided. Occasionally a haemorrhage into the cerebellum is diagnosed and this benefits from surgical drainage. How much influence these differences in management have on prognosis has not yet been quantified, but most GPs addressing this question felt that all patients with stroke who enjoy a good quality of life and who do not appear to be terminally ill require the benefit of a scan.

5 A Siriraj score of >12, calculated as shown below from evidence obtained around 24 h after hospital admission for stroke, indicates a probable haemorrhage. Such patients have high priority for a scan to confirm the haemorrhage, as neurosurgery may improve the prognosis.

Consciousness	Alert	0	
	Drowsy	2.5	
	Semicoma	5.0	____
+ Vomiting	No	0	
	Yes	2	____
+ Headache within 2 h of onset	No	0	
	Yes	2	____
+ Diastolic blood pressure in mmHg divided by 10			____
+ One or more of the following: diabetes, ischaemic heart disease and intermittent claudication	No	0	
	Yes	3	____
		Total	____

Similar observations when the patient is first seen may be valuable in deciding whether the patient should be admitted as a matter of urgency for a brain scan.

6 Stroke rehabilitation units have a good record for improving mortality and quality of life of stroke patients. The work of physiotherapists, occupational therapists and speech therapists is greatly eased by having the patients attend these therapists at their place of work. Unfortunately, provision of these units is patchy, and in their absence the work of therapists, nurses and social carers is often poorly co-ordinated, with no one taking effective overall responsibility.

GPs addressing this question mentioned in particular the need for effective medical responsibility and day-to-day attendance by a well-informed and well-supported carer.

They also mentioned some specific facilities that are sometimes neglected. These are listed below.

- Carers and nurses need to be well informed about positioning the patient in order to limit the risk of contractures, and about the measures they can take to maximize the patient's independence.

- Mobility aids include a chair from which the patient can rise, as well as grab rails and hoists by the bedside and bath. Trolleys and walking sticks with tripod feet are used more than Zimmer aids.

- Occasional visits from a community psychiatric nurse may help to prevent depression, or lead to its earlier recognition.

- Voluntary support groups may provide a visitor for company and advocacy, and help with correspondence and occasional outings.

- Patients who can take advantage of a mobility allowance to obtain an adapted car and an orange parking badge from the local authority need to be told of these benefits.

- A dietitian may attend in order to advise on the use of convenience foods which the patient can prepare personally.

- Co-ordination of these services may be helped if all who attend make entries in a patient-held record file.

- Carers need to be told whom to contact in order to arrange respite care and changes in the services to cope with altered needs.

7 The writer of the original article recommended analysing the situation of patients who require rehabilitation into strengths and weaknesses, and setting both short-term and medium-term targets. GPs addressing this question considered that it might be worth mentioning the following points in particular in discussion.

- The couple would be spending more time together. Would they like to read about how to develop their relationship, or discuss this either with the doctor or with a Relate counsellor?

- Having stopped smoking and excessive drinking and controlled other risk factors, Robert is at a much reduced risk of stroke recurrence.

- Robert will have more time to be with his grandchildren and can now pursue new hobbies.

  Targets within the next week might include the following.

- Difficulty in chopping food could be helped immediately by using a Nelson combined knife and fork.
- An elbow crutch and a commode, and a grab handle above the bed and the armchair could enable Robert to be more mobile and independent immediately.
- The Citizens Advice Bureau and the DSS and Building Society could advise on rearranging finances. The couple should bear in mind that the local authority would find it cheaper for them to stay where they are than to rehouse them.
- Robert could chart his progress in increasing his mobility and dexterity at tasks around the house.
- The couple could arrange a regular daily time for discussion of how to face the future together.
- Dial-a-Ride could provide transport at low cost.

  Longer-term targets might include the following.

- Support could be organized from a local day centre and community physiotherapists, occupational therapists and volunteer carers.
- Robert could be assessed for his ability to drive an adapted car provided that he has normal visual fields and no anosognosia.
- Directories of holidays for the disabled could be consulted.

8 a False.

   b False – up to 50% of fit elderly people have no gag reflex, and the absence of a gag reflex after a stroke does not indicate either inability to swallow or the presence of aspiration.

9 a True.

   b False – it requires sedation and local anaesthetic only.

THERAPEUTICS

Gastrointestinal effects

1 What drug treatment is most likely to be effective for nausea and vomiting due to the following conditions?

  a Introduction of opioids.

  b Cytotoxic chemotherapy.

  c Renal failure.

  d Inoperable gastroduodenal obstruction.

  e Raised intracranial pressure.

  f Vestibular disturbance.

  g Bowel obstruction.

  BMJ. **315**: 1148–50

2 What form of cancer may be prevented by taking aspirin regularly?

  BMJ. **304**: 62

Cardiovascular effects

1 ACE inhibitors: (*True/False*)

  a may cause a fall in glomerular filtration rate for several weeks when first introduced

  b necessitate monitoring of serum potassium in patients with renal impairment

  c are dangerous for patients with renal artery stenosis.

  BMJ. **304**: 327–8

2 Why may high-dose enalapril tablets provoke an allergic reaction when low-dose ones do not.

BMJ. **311**: 1204 (drug points)

3 With which drugs and medical conditions may terfenadine interact to produce QT prolongation and a danger of arrhythmia? (*5 points*)

BMJ. **314**: 248 (news item)

4 Which drugs are liable to interact with cisapride to produce a prolonged QT interval and susceptibility to ventricular arrhythmia? (*4 points*)

BMJ. **316**: 101 (news item)

Central nervous system effects

1 What psychosocial factors may account for the placebo effect, and how can they be used in order to maximize it? (*4 or more points*)

BMJ. **311**: 1640

2 You are substituting another route of administration for oral morphine. What proportional change in the total daily dose is likely to be needed:

a for rectal administration

b for subcutaneous administration

c for intravenous administration?

BMJ. **312**: 823–6

3 What two types of drug may exacerbate the reaction to an insect sting?

BMJ. **305**: 946

4 Should on-call doctors in the community carry a vial of flumazenil in their bags? Give two reasons for your point of view.

BMJ. **301**: 1308–11

5 What symptomatic side-effects can be expected in most patients starting treatment with high doses of oral steroids? (*2 points*)

BMJ. **306**: 1477–8

6 There is evidence that the following are effective therapies: (*True/False*)

a sodium valproate for migraine

b prednisolone for herpes zoster

c carbamazepine for herpes zoster.

BMJ. **311**: 1047–52 (review)

---

7 Ten milligrams of diazepam are equivalent to how many milligrams of the following benzodiazepines?

a Chlordiazepoxide.

b Temazepam.

c Nitrazepam.

d Lorazepam.

BMJ. **315**: 297–300 (review)

---

8 Zopiclone may cause physical dependence. (*True/False*)

BMJ. **316**: 117 (case reports)

---

9 Temazepam 10 mg nocte has been found to aggravate sleep apnoea in climbers adjusting to altitude. (*True/False)*

BMJ. **316**: 587–9 (research report)

---

10 Paracetamol overdose.

a What factors enhance the toxicity of paracetamol?

b What reporting error may explain toxicity occurring even when paracetamol levels have been lower than the danger line?

BMJ. **316**: 1295–8 (review)
BMJ. **316**: 1724–5 (case reports)

---

11 What is the maximal daily dose of oral paracetamol recommended for children?

BMJ. **316**: 1552 (leading article)

---

12 You are starting a 70 kg adult on lithium to prevent mood swings.

a What initial dose will you use?

b When will you ask him to come back to check the serum level?

c What type of container will you use for the sample and what other precaution will you take?

d Assuming the result is in the therapeutic range, what advice will you give the patient to follow thereafter?

BMJ. **305**: 1273–6
BMJ. **306**: 269–70

Miscellaneous

1   What medicinal uses are there for chewing gum? (*3 or more points*)

BMJ. **313**:1180–4 (research report)

2   What seems to offer the best protection against biting midges? (*1 point*)

BMJ. **313**:1216 (citation)

3   What key events should patients on anticoagulants bring to the attention of the person responsible for supervising their anticoagulant care? (*5 points*)

BMJ. **312**: 286 (research report)

4   Rebound salt and water retention may occur if diuretics are stopped suddenly. (*True/False*)

BMJ. **316**: 628 (letter)

5   Which medicines are known to cause muscle cramps? (*7 points*)

BMJ. **306**: 1169

BMJ. **311**: 1541 (short research report)

6   Which drugs have been shown to reduce bone loss in patients requiring long-term oral prednisolone? (*2 points*)

BMJ. **307**: 519–20

7   What drug may be useful for pruritus associated with cholestasis of pregnancy?

BMJ. **312**: 1430 (citation)

8   What advantage may there be in giving thrombolytic drugs by catheter in the treatment of DVT?

BMJ. **312**: 1430 (citation)

9   Trials in a single subject involve randomly alternating active and placebo treatment under double-blind conditions in order to determine whether improvement coincides with the use of active treatment. List three or more conditions in which this 'suck it and see' approach to therapy might be justified.

BMJ. **303**: 173–4

10 Patients taking the following drugs are at particular risk of hyponatraemia: (*True/False*)

a a thiazide diuretic

b diazepam

c a macrolide antibiotic

d allopurinol

e an antineoplastic agent.

BMJ. **307**: 305–8 (review)

11 The bone-marrow toxicity of chloramphenicol is known to be dose related. (*True/False*)

BMJ. **310**: 1217–18

12 What rare serious side-effects seem to be much more common with minocycline than with tetracycline? (*4 points*)

BMJ. **312**: 138 (review)

13 What inhalation may help blood to clot in a bleeding patient?

BMJ. **315**: 1320 (citation)

14 What are the likely medicinal uses of marijuana? (*4 or more points*)

BMJ. **315**: 504

15 What may be the true medical indications for thalidomide? (*4 points*)

BMJ. **315**: 699 (news item)

16 What are the currently accepted indications for massive intravenous doses of polyvalent immunoglobulin? (*6 or more points*)

BMJ. **312**: 1465–8 (review)

17 What dangers are associated with infusions of polyvalent gammaglobulin for autoimmune conditions? (*5 points*)

BMJ. **315**:1203–4 (case report and comment)

18 Certain drugs are excreted in fetotoxic amounts in semen and should not be used by men who are having unprotected intercourse with fertile women. Which drugs are they?

BMJ. **312**: 1053–4 (review)

ANSWERS

Gastrointestinal effects

1 a Introduction of opioids – metoclopramide 30–80 mg/24 h or haloperidol 1.5–10 mg/24 h.

   b Cytotoxic chemotherapy – 5–HT$_3$ antagonists such as ondansetron. High-dose metoclopramide and dexamethasone may be effective. Benzodiazepines may reduce anticipatory anxiety and thus prevent vomiting.

   c Renal failure – haloperidol.

   d Inoperable gastroduodenal obstruction – metoclopramide, dexamethasone, octreotide.

   e Raised intracranial pressure – dexamethasone 8–20 mg/24 h.

   f Vestibular disturbance – cyclizine 150 mg/24 h or sublingual or transdermal hyoscine hydrobromide.

   g Bowel obstruction – haloperidol, cyclizine, methotrimeprazine 12.5–75 mg/24 h, hyoscine butylbromide 60–300 mg/24 h, octreotide 300–600 mcg/24 h.

2 Cancer of the colon.

Cardiovascular effects

1 a True.

   b True.

   c True.

2 High-dose enalapril tablets (10 mg and 20 mg) contain the colouring agents mapico red or mapico yellow. Low-dose tablets (2.5 mg and 5 mg) are free of colouring.

3 Erythromycin, clarithromycin, ketoconazole and itraconazole, and in liver disease.

4 Macrolide antibiotics, antifungals, some antidepressants, and protease inhibitors. Cisapride is also contraindicated if there is hypokalaemia, chronic obstructive airways disease, congestive heart failure or advanced cancer. Patients taking insulin, and those with gastrointestinal disturbance or dehydration, are also warned against taking cisapride.

Central nervous system effects

1 The placebo effect appears to be related to the patient's need to understand and control the illness, and to build hope, self-esteem and a sense of being in rational control of the problem. In order to maximize the effect we need to share lay and medical understanding and build concordance with patients, confidence in the prescriber and confidence in the capacity of the patient to experience alleviation of the illness.

2 a No change.

 b Halve the dose.

 c Reduce the dose to one third.

3 Beta-blockers and NSAIDs.

4 Flumazenil is an antidote to benzodiazepines in overdose. GPs' answers could be summarized as follows.

 Yes, on-call doctors should carry flumazenil because:
 • it is of proven efficacy in the diagnosis of coma due to self-poisoning
 • it precludes the need for numerous other therapeutic procedures in some patients.

 No, on-call doctors should not carry flumazenil because:
 • it would rarely be required by the individual doctor
 • it is best given under conditions of continuous supervision.

5 Insomnia and bad dreams. However, asthmatics do not seem to complain much about these problems, which are perhaps restricted to cancer sufferers.

6 a True – 25 out of 29 cases found it effective at a dose of 400 mg bd. On average it reduced the frequency of attacks by roughly 50% and the intensity by about 40%.

 b True – skin healed significantly faster with prednisolone (40 mg/day for 10 days, then tailed off over the next 3 weeks) than with carbamazepine, and the incidence of post-herpetic neuralgia was 3/20 in the prednisolone group and 13/20 in the carbamazepine group.

 c False – see above.

7 a 30 mg.

 b 20 mg.

 c 10 mg.

 d 1 mg.

8 True – case reports are presented.

9 False – at this low dose it improved it.

10 a Chronic alcohol misuse, eating disorders, enzyme-inducing drugs.

 b Concealment of the real time of overdose or the number of tablets taken.

11 An upper limit of 90 mg/kg/day and a loading dose of 30 mg/kg are becoming accepted.

12 a 400–600 mg/day in two doses.

    b 12 h after dosing 1 week later.

    c No anticoagulant in the sample tube.

    d • Do not take water tablets or anti-inflammatory tablets such as aspirin unless the doctor who is prescribing them is aware that you are taking lithium.

        • Avoid becoming dehydrated, particularly if you suffer a gastric upset. Reduce the dose of lithium or seek medical advice if you suffer prolonged diarrhoea or vomiting.

        • Tremor, thirst, some weight gain and some diarrhoea are natural effects of the drug and are not signs that it is causing you any harm.

        • Recheck serum lithium levels, thyroid function and urea and electrolytes after 3 months, and periodically thereafter.

Miscellaneous

1 • It prevents caries and otitis media if it contains xylitol rather than sucrose.

   • It increases saliva flow, so helps xerostomia and halitosis and neutralizes acid reflux from the stomach and can thus help to control heartburn.

   • It can be used as an aid to dieting and a substitute for tobacco.

   • It can serve as a displacement activity for anxious people.

2 Oil of bog myrtle (*Myrica gale*).

3 A change in any other treatment, any bruising or bleeding, any visit to casualty, any admission to hospital, and any impending surgery or dentistry in the next 2 months.

4 True – so either stop them gradually or, better still, advise patients to reduce their salt intake.

5 Beta-two agonists, steroids (including inhaled steroids), diuretics, danazol, nifedipine, cimetidine, and laxatives if they cause dehydration.

6 Pamidronate and calcitriol.

7 Ondansetron – a serotonin receptor antagonist.

8 This reduces the incidence of post-thrombotic syndrome, but it may increase the risk of pulmonary embolism.

9 Trials that involve alternating active and placebo treatment at random intervals could be useful for determining an individual patient's responsiveness to treatment. One practical problem is finding identical placebos to branded medicines without invoking the help of the manufacturer, who will be influenced by legal and commercial considerations. Vitamin or health-food tablets may have to suffice for the placebo treatment.

Doctors addressing this question suggested that such trials might be useful in the differential diagnosis of symptoms which may or may not be of physical origin, e.g using GTN tablets in the diagnosis of angina in a patient with vague chest symptoms, or identifying whether headache or limb pain are genuinely responsive to analgesics or NSAIDs, whether abdominal pain is responsive to antisecretory or antispasmodic drugs, whether neuralgia responds to low-dose amitriptyline, whether headache responds to sumatriptan or its congeners, or whether urinary urgency responds to detrusor stabilizers.

10 **a** True.

  b True.

  c False.

  d False.

  e True.

11 False – there have been reports of fatal idiosyncratic pancytopenic reactions to ocular chloramphenicol drops, as well as the reversible dose-related suppression of the erythroid cell line which occurs at very high oral doses.

12 Chronic active hepatitis, eosinophilic pneumonitis, systemic lupus erythematosus and arthralgia.

13 Desmopressin.

14 To treat anorexia in cancer and AIDS, nausea and vomiting while on cancer chemotherapy, muscle spasm in multiple sclerosis, and to reduce eyeball pressure in glaucoma.

15 Inflammation associated with leprosy, some cancers, lupus, graft-versus-host disease, and some complications of AIDS.

16 Idiopathic thrombocytopenic purpura, Kawasaki disease, steroid-resistant dermatomyositis, and possibly selected cases of haemophilia, intractable asthma, myasthenia gravis, Guillain-Barré syndrome, systemic lupus erythematosus and primary phospholipid syndrome.

17 Aseptic meningitis starting 6–48 h after infusion and lasting up to 5 days has an incidence of 11–17%.

  Common side-effects include headache, fever, chills and nausea. Rare, more serious side-effects are anaphylaxis, haemolysis, hepatitis and thrombosis.

18 Griseofulvin and finasteride.

TUBERCULOSIS

1 How does the British Thoracic Society recommend that close contacts of an open case of TB be screened?

BMJ. **304**: 1213–15 (case report)
BMJ. **313**: 221–2 (case report)

2 An African patient in the UK has TB. What proportion of such patients are likely to be HIV positive?

BMJ. **314**: 1747–50 (review)

3 Which immigrants should a GP refer to the local chest clinic to exclude TB?

BMJ. **307**: 1539–40

4 What are the likely presentations of abdominal TB? (*2 points*)

BMJ. **315**: 1388 (citation)

5 *Mycobacterium paratuberculosis.* (*True/False*)

a It is found in milk from affected cattle.

b It is always sensitive to pasteurization.

c It causes chronic granulomatous inflammation in the human intestine.

d It causes a positive Mantoux test.

e DNA detection from biopsy samples is the best means to establish the diagnosis.

f Many months of treatment with antibiotics effective against this organism may also cure Crohn's disease.

BMJ. **316**: 449–53 (case report)

ANSWERS

1 For patients under 16 years of age, Heaf test; for those aged 16–50 years, Heaf test plus chest X-ray; for those aged over 50 years, chest X-ray. However, some authorities suggest that children under 16 years of age should also have a chest X-ray.

2 19%.

3 Only a tiny minority of immigrants have open TB, but a recent letter in the *BMJ* reveals that a significant percentage are either tuberculin negative, or are children with strongly positive results on tuberculin testing that justify chemoprophylaxis. An active policy of screening and treatment is therefore justified for any immigrant who has relevant symptoms, or who has no evidence of previous tuberculin testing.

4 Ascites and diarrhoea.

5 a True.
   b False.
   c True – together with lymphadenopathy and arthritis in some cases.
   d True.
   e True – it is rarely cultured from the human intestine, and when it is cultured it is usually in a non-bacillary form.
   f True – rifabutin and clarithromycin.

URINARY INFECTION

1 What should a female patient do while urinating to reduce the likelihood that a sample of urine that she provides for bacteriology is contaminated with surface organisms?

Br J Gen Pract. **42**: 241–3

2 When using urine collection pads to obtain samples from infants or incontinent confused, elderly people, what instructions should be given to the supervisor?

Br J Gen Pract. **48**: 1342–3 (letter)

3 How can you test for urethritis in a sexually active man? What will you do if the test is positive?

BMJ. **313**: 112 (correspondence)

4 What is the probability of significant bacteriuria in a urine sample from a patient with suspected UTI which is clear to the eye and negative for blood, protein and nitrite on dipstick testing?

Br J Gen Pract. **42**: 36, 346–7

BMJ. **306**: 1512

5 What factors may predispose to a false-negative result on dipstick tests for leucocyte esterase? (*5 points*)

BMJ. **313**: 1009–10 (letter)

6 What artefact may clavulanic acid cause in urine test-strip results?

BMJ. **313**: 25 (research report)

7 What sampling and testing factors influence the sensitivity of the nitrite test to nitrite-producing bacteria in the urine?

Br J Gen Pract. **43**: 37

8 Urine infections in infants. (*True/False*)

  a About 1 in 12 hospitalized infants with unexplained fever or serious illness have bacteriuria.

  b More than 100 000 organisms/mL is a useful standard when screening infants' suprapubic aspirates for bacteriuria.

  c About 50% of infants with bacteriuria have abnormalities on investigation of the urinary tract.

  d A negative ultrasound scan in infants with bacteriuria obviates the need for further investigation.

BMJ. **308**: 690–2

9 A 4-year-old child has fever and dysuria.

  a How would you obtain and transmit a urine specimen to the laboratory?

  b If the result showed significant bacteriuria, what further investigations and follow-up would you arrange?

  c If further investigation revealed renal scarring, what further follow-up or treatment would you expect or arrange? (*2 points*)

BMJ. **301**: 301

10 Urinary tract infections: (*True/False*)

  a in elderly men are almost certainly due to Enterobacteriaceae

  b only rarely provoke dipstick haematuria

  c may be due to candida in patients with catheters

  d in pregnancy should be treated with a prolonged (7–14 day) course of treatment.

BMJ. **305**:1137–41

11 What further investigations would you arrange for the following patients with sterile pyuria?

  a A sexually active young man with a painless urethral discharge.

  b A post-menopausal woman with dysuria who occasionally has intercourse with her husband.

Br J Gen Pract. **44**: 114–17

12 What errors do doctors commonly make when discussing risk factors for urinary infection with female patients?

Br J Gen Pract. **48**: 1155–7 (interview survey report)

13 Cranberry juice drink, 300 mL/day, taken as prophylaxis or treatment for recurrent urinary tract infections in elderly women can be expected to: (*True/False*)

a reduce the incidence of first attacks of UTI significantly

b reduce the prevalence of UTI significantly

c improve the resolution of UTI significantly.

BMJ. **312**: 364–7 (citation)

4 What measures, in addition to a prescription for a short course of antibiotic, may help a 70-year-old woman who suffers recurrent cystitis?

BMJ. **313**: 129 (leading article)

ANSWERS

1 Hold the labia apart.

2 Pads should be checked every 10 to 20 min in babies. The urine is withdrawn with a syringe, and can be placed in a universal container which is kept in a refrigerator. They are available from NHS stores (Order No. CFQ 152).

3 The two-glass test. The first 40–50 mL of urine are caught in the first container, and the residuum is collected in the second. If the patient has urethritis, the first container will be turbid and the second one will be clear. If the test is positive, the patient should be tested for *Neisseria gonorrhoeae* and *Chlamydia trachomatis*. *Chlamydia* may be missed unless some time is allowed to elapse between urination and taking the swab.

4 2–5%.

5 Approximately 9% of such tests have been found to be false negatives. Most such false-negative results were obtained in patients taking antibiotics, while the others were in patients with ketonuria and glycosuria.

6 A false-positive result for leucocyte esterase.

7 The time interval since previous micturition, and the time period permitted for a colour change to develop.

8 a True.
  b False.
  c True.
  d False.

9 a Clean the end of the penis with a wet tissue or cloth which does not have antiseptic or disinfectant added. Ask the child to pass a little urine into the toilet, and then a little into the urine container. If the container contains no preservative, ensure that it reaches the laboratory within 2 h during working hours, or that it is kept in the refrigerator until it is transported to the laboratory.
  b Ultrasound or IVP to demonstrate whether there are anatomical abnormalities, ureteric reflux or renal scars. Repeat the MSU after a course of antibiotic.
  c Surgical management or long-term antibiotics if a ureteric reflux is found. Regular follow-up with MSUs to ensure that urine is kept free of infection if no reflux is found.

10 a False – 39% are due to Gram-positive organisms.
   b False – 50% of cases.
   c True.
   d True.

11 a Test the urine for chlamydial antigen, and take a urethral swab for chlamydial culture and neisserial culture.

b Test the urine for chlamydial antigen, and take cervical and urethral swabs for chlamydial culture and neisserial culture.

12 • Failing to mention that sexual intercourse is a common precipitating factor. Only 39% of the women in this survey were aware of this risk factor.

• Talking about a short urethra, and giving women the impression that they are deformed compared to others of the same sex.

• Failing to mention the diaphragm as a precipitating cause in women who use this method of contraception.

• Failing to correct the widespread impression among women that tight clothing and the use of bubble bath are risk factors.

13 a False – in this study, 10.2 first events per 100 person months in the treatment group compared to 12.5 first events per 100 person months in the placebo group.

b True – in this study, 15% of monthly samples tested positive in the treatment group, compared to 28% in the placebo group.

c True – in this study, the probability of change from positive to negative in 1 month was 0.54 in the treatment group, compared to 0.28 in the placebo group.

14 Base longer-term antibiotic treatment on culture results, including culture for fastidious organisms such as *Ureaplasma urealyticum* and *Mycoplasma hominis*, and use oestrogen cream. If this is unsuccessful, perform a pelvic examination, cystoscopy and bladder biopsy and urodynamics. If symptoms occur after intercourse, use vaginal lubricant and a prophylactic antibiotic.

Cystoscopy and biopsy may identify interstitial cystitis by increased mast-cell count. This may benefit from hexamine hippurate 1 g bd or a tricyclic antidepressant or prednisolone 15 mg/day during month 1, 10 mg/day during month 2, and 5 mg/day during month 3.